Laughter Exercises:
The Great Big Anthology

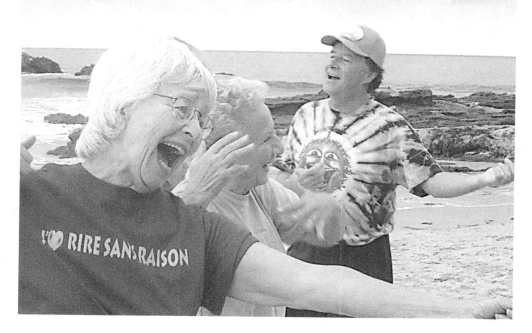

Photo-illustrated

Five hundred laughter practices
for health, fun and friendship

**Includes Dr. Kataria's Foundation Exercises,
Laughter/Breathing Techniques, and Laughter Meditation**

Compiled, edited and written by Jeffrey Briar
with numerous contributors

Black-&-White Edition – Revised & Updated 2016

In two sections:
> **Part 1: Dr. Kataria's Foundation Exercises**
> **Part 2: Encyclopedia of Laughter Exercises**

At The Laughter Yoga Institute, we take laughter seriously.

Laughter Exercises: The Great Big Anthology

(with 120 photographs)

Black-&-White edition of
"The Great Big Anthology of Laughter Exercises" (2011, revised 2017)

By Jeffrey Briar

ISBN-13: 978-1533456328

ISBN 10: 1533456321

Published in the USA by
Creative Arts Press
790 Manzanita Drive
Laguna Beach, California 92651
(949) 376-1939   info@LYInstitute.org

Table of Contents

Illustration credits:
p. 67 &c., p. 121 : Lynn Kubasek
p. 103 : Jamian Briar
P. 104 : David Fleischmann

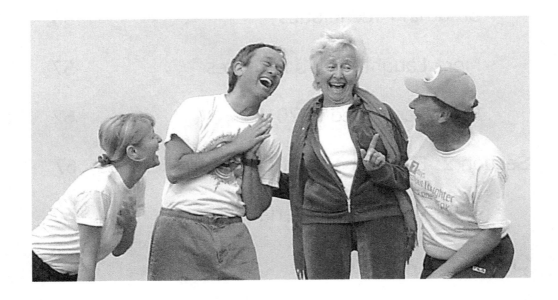

Laguna Laughter Club Staff

Laughing daily by the sea since 2005

Kathryn Burns, Jeffrey Briar, Ruthe Gluckson, David Sullenger

Laughter as Exercise

Here are simple, *free* activities to bring you more joy, new friends, and better health; an abundance of laugh-evoking practices for use at Laughter Clubs, starters for Improv theatre games, or for any declared "playtime" for people of all ages. More fun than a pile of puppies, as much joy as finding buried pirate treasure… such are the delights you'll find from this cheerful book.

What is "Laughter as Exercise"?

Sometimes called Laughter Yoga, this is a technique of producing laughter for its own sake without the need for jokes or comedy. Participants interact playfully like children having fun together at a playground. Thanks to the social interaction the laughter quickly becomes genuine and heartfelt.

Laughter Yoga was created in India in 1995 by Dr. Madan Kataria, a medical doctor, in collaboration with his wife Madhuri, a yoga teacher. The first Laughter Club consisted of five people in a park in Bombay (Mumbai). Hundreds of thousands of people worldwide now practice laughter for health.

A typical laughter session includes: easy stretches, breathing practices, and an assortment of intentional laughter techniques such as those you will find in this collection. The exercises are simple and very pleasant to perform. There is no need for costly equipment, mats, or special clothing. Participants choose their level of engagement, from gentle to vigorous. The experience is suitable for all ages and all levels of ability. Laughing classmates tend to form caring, supportive friendships. Participants live life more joyfully and find themselves better able to cope with whatever stresses life may bring them.

Why laugh?

In the 1960s journalist Norman Cousins cured himself of a painful terminal disease through the use of alternative therapies which included his watching a steady supply of funny movies and TV shows. His book *Anatomy of an Illness – as Perceived by the Patient* led to extensive medical research.

Some of the reported Benefits of Laughter include:

- Relieves stress - reduces adrenaline and cortisol
- Reduces anxiety, fear, depression - raises serotonin levels
- Enhances the immune system - boosts natural anti-viral and anti-cancer cell activity
- Improves respiratory and cardiovascular systems - dilates blood vessels, balances blood pressure; increases lung capacity, increases oxygen levels in blood and brain
- Relieves pain - produces an endorphin-like effect: the "Biochemistry of Happiness"
- Encourages relaxation of muscles and mind
- Boosts self-confidence, promotes compassion, deepens creativity

To achieve significant health effects, laughter needs to be of sufficient duration. Most studies declare 10 to 20 minutes are required to achieve the desirable physiological changes. An occasional chuckle does not lead to the best results. Jokes and comedy are not reliable sources for generating laughter lasting such a length of time, but Laughter as Exercise can dependably do the job. The practice of intentional laughter also develops our sense of humor: we find ourselves more likely to find things amusing, and are able to see the lighter, brighter side of life. Thanks to the discovery and development of this kind of Laughter Without Jokes *you need never be stressed-out again*.

Laughter for your life

Laughter activities are practical, popular additions to yoga classes, at senior centers, and for business meetings. Students have more fun, are less self-critical, and develop more friendships. They feel less pain and are more outgoing. Class attendance goes up. Laughter "breaks" during meetings and study sessions result in more focused attention, better retention and greater involvement. Laughter in the workplace leads to employees who are genuinely happy to go to work every day.

About this book

This publication attempts to be comprehensive in offering practical laughter exercises, but only hints at the history and theory behind Laughter Yoga. For a more comprehensive discussion of the Laughter Yoga story and philosophy please see *The Laughter Yoga Book* by Jeffrey Briar and/or *Laugh for No Reason* by Dr. Madan Kataria.

How to Lead a Laughter Exercise

All sessions are preceded with the advice that students can participate at whatever energy level they wish. They are welcome to modify any practice to suit their personal comfort level, or refrain from performing any activity which they think might cause them discomfort.

The Three "D's" - Declare, Demonstrate, and Do (Alternatively: "Say; Show; 'Go!'")

Step 1: *Declare* (Denote/De-name) (or "**Say**"). Say the name of the exercise.

> "The next exercise is called 'Penguin Laughter.'"

Step 2: *Demonstrate* (or "**Show**"). Show physically how to perform the exercise, while simultaneously verbalizing the instruction.

> "Start with your feet turned out [*place your feet in this position:*], arms straight down by your sides, hands flexed, palms facing the floor. Walk around like a penguin [*do a stiff-legged walk, the upward-flexed hands swinging into and then away from the legs*]. Play with or follow behind the other penguins, laughing all the while [*make eye contact with other participants, lean towards them in greeting*]."

Step 3: *Do* (or "'**Go!**'"). First: stop the demonstration. Then: give a clear "Command to Start." This is done with a sense of building up tension such that everyone will release into laughing together, all at the same time, the moment you give them the cue to do so.

> "Okay, 'got your feet turned out? Ready – set: *Go!*" (immediately burst into laughter).
> > Or: "Penguins, are you ready? *Take off!*"
> > Or: "Here we go: One, two, three, *Waddle!*"

Allow the exercise to run for at least 15 seconds - 30 to 45 seconds is preferred. Some enthusiastic groups may run an entire minute or longer. (In some countries, each laughter exercise may be run for two to five minutes!) Tune in to your group: allow for space wherein participants can go beyond their initial effort of copying the Leader and get to where they explore nuances and discover their own creative impulses.

Conclude the exercise by calling out words of praise (like **"Great job, everyone!"** - also see "Encouraging Words", available from www.LYInstitute.org) or doing the **"Ho, ho, ha-ha-ha"** (p. 57) or **"Very good, very good, Yay!"** practice (p. 60).

There are numerous examples available for viewing on YouTube. Please visit our accounts under "JoyfulGent" and "Jeffrey Briar" or search under "laughter exercise briar".

We hope you enjoy your adventure into the joyous, playful world of Laughter as Exercise. Laughter encourages imagination; watch yourself create your own new exercises! Laughter Clubs welcome all participants and new ideas, so let yourself experience the delight of your Laughter Club members bringing in and making up new laughter exercises which you can share with the world. You can share laughter exercises, as well as getting laughter-related advice and leadership coaching, through our free online group "Laugh4Health" on YahooGroups.

Joyful Be!

-- Jeffrey Briar

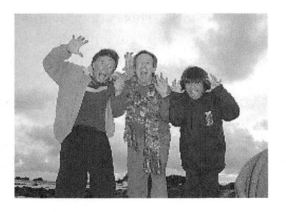

Part 1

Doctor Kataria's Foundation Exercises

Sixty-plus Doctor-recommended Laughter Exercises used by Laughter Clubs all over the world

Black-&-White Version
Revised & Updated 2017

The Laughter Yoga Institute

www.LYInstitute.org

This volume is a support tool for Laughter Exercise Leaders. The practices are those which Dr. Kataria, creator of Laughter Yoga, requested be taught at all training programs worldwide from 2006-2015. Exercises added by Dr. Kataria in 2015 are on pp. 62-64. Once you are familiar with these exercises you will share a common body of knowledge – as well as friendship - with Laughter Exercise Leaders all over the planet.

The exercises are provided in alphabetical order A to Z. There are additional Laughter and Breathing Exercises in the end portion of this section. The images were originally solicited to support the Laughter Exercise Photo Flash Cards (these are out-of-print, but you can order files to make your own cards via www.laughter-exercise-cards.info; on this website there are also translations of the exercises into several languages). Laughter lovers from 23 countries are represented.

All exercises are performed "while laughing." The numbers following each description indicate the level of vigorousness typically associated with the exercise. Low numbers (1-3) signify a gentle practice; high numbers (8-10) are more energetically expressed. Even so, laughers are encouraged to participate at whatever level feels comfortable for them.

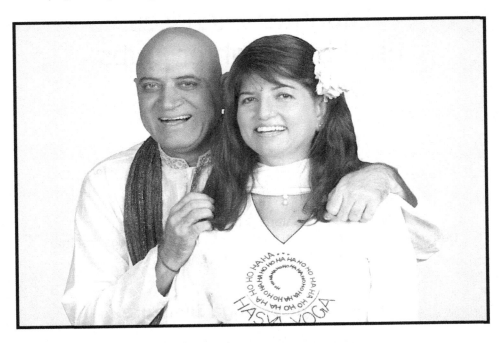

Dr. Madan and Mrs. Madhuri Kataria

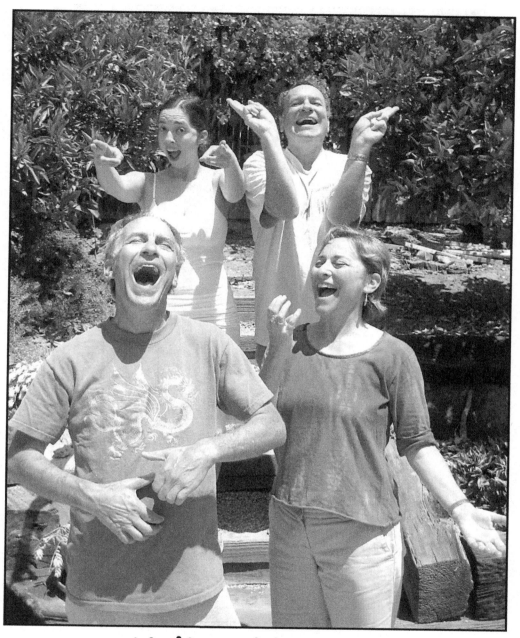

Airline Hostess

Demonstrate: 1. Where to find the emergency exits and floor lighting. 2. How to operate the seatbelt. 3. Pull down oxygen mask; put on self, then another. 4. Inflate life jacket (blowing into tube). 4 – 7

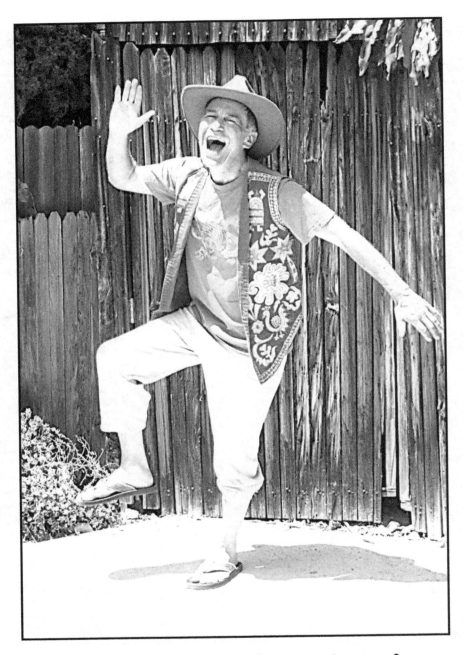

American (Cowboy)

Slap the thighs, one or both like a cowboy from the Wild West). Raise up your big hat, "Yee-haw;" place fists on hips, ride a horse, twirl six guns. Big, broad, roaring laughs: "Hardy har har!" 4 – 9 [Omitted 2015]

12

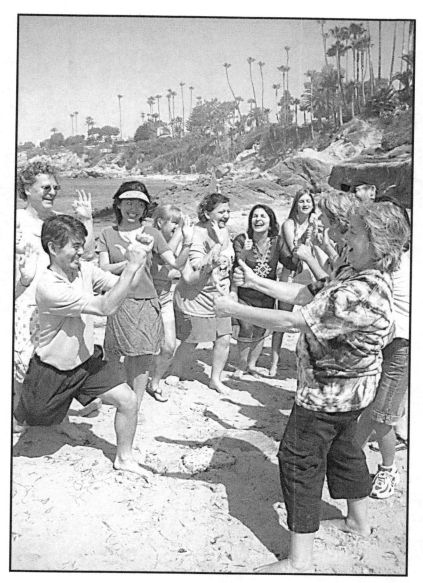

Appreciation
(Acknowledgment)

Bring the tip of the index finger to meet the tip of the
thumb to make a small circle: "O-kay!" or use a "thumbs-
up" gesture. Walk around expressing appreciation: "Ah-
ha-ha, great job!" "Well done!" "Alright!" Can applaud
briefly, throw kisses, "give me five", etc. 2 - 5

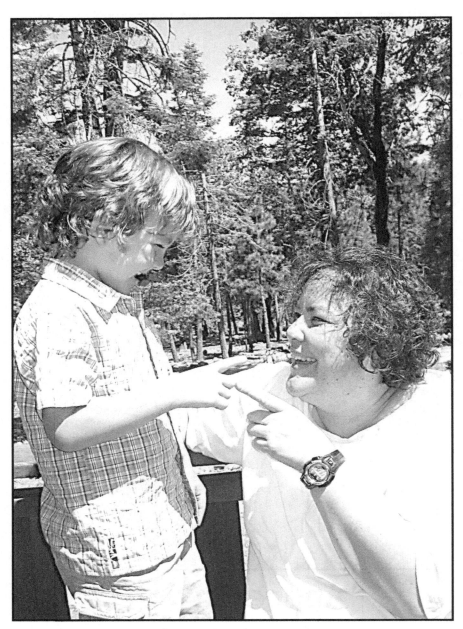

Argument
(Naughty-Naughty)

Pretend to "argue" by pointing and waggling index
fingers at each other. Playful only, nothing serious!
(Follow with "Forgiveness" p. 25)   4 – 8

14

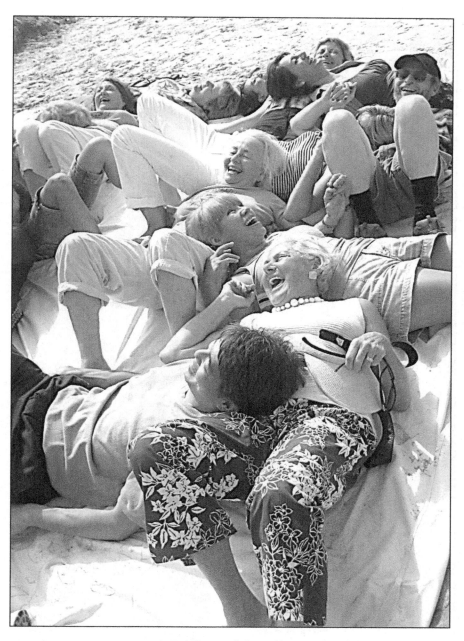

Belly
(Head On The Belly)

Lie down at right angles with your head on another's
belly, and someone else's head on your belly. 3 – 7

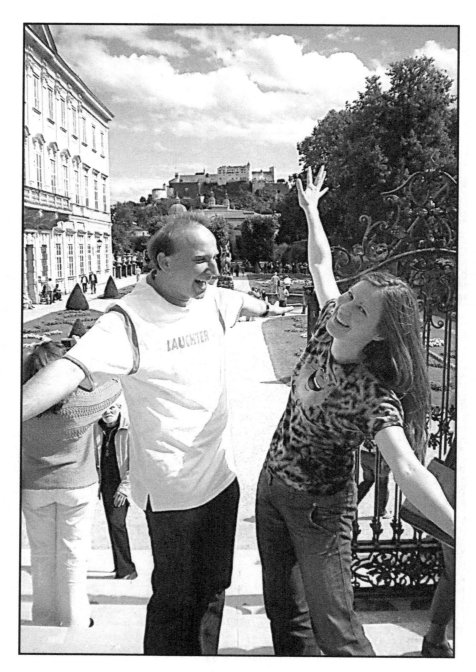

Bird

Extend your arms like a bird; flap "wings," take off, drift
and fly - all different directions.   5 – 8

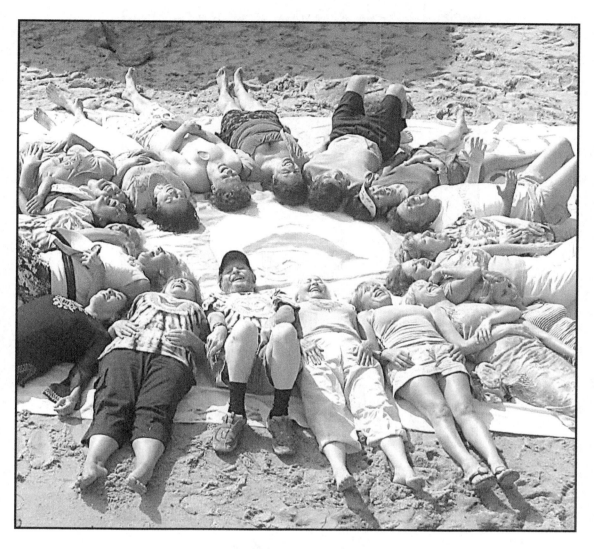

Bullseye
(Sunflower, Target)

Lie on the back, heads towards the center of the circle, feet out towards the periphery (looking like the petals of a flower, the spokes of a wheel, or a target). Do "Laughter Meditation" (eyes closed, laughing for no reason, see p. 58) or "Centipede" (p. 20) exercises. 2 – 9

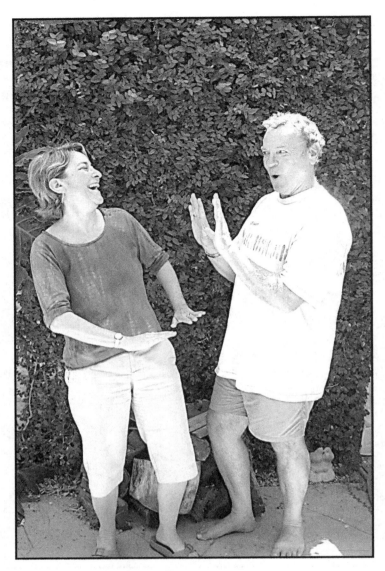

Calcutta

Everyone does simultaneously. Hands in front: two short sharp repetitions of "Ho, Ho" with hands pushing forward; follow with two repetitions of "Ha, Ha" with hands facing down and pushing sharply downwards. Include a slight bounce in the knees; can do dance-like movements, hands to one side, above the head, etc. Repeat for 15 to 30 seconds. Can speed up; allow to turn into free, unregulated laughter. 7 – 10 [Omitted 2015]

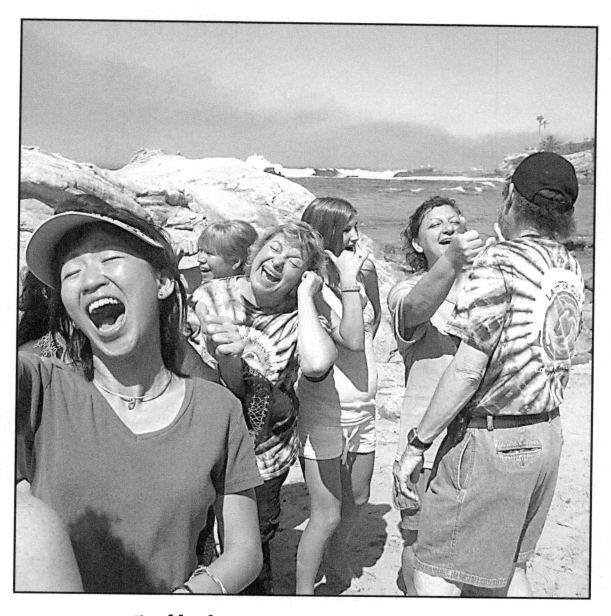

Cellphone (Mobilephone)

Hold an imaginary cell phone; put it to your ear; laugh at
what you hear. Move around and share with others;
they laugh at your cellphone, you laugh at theirs.   4 – 6

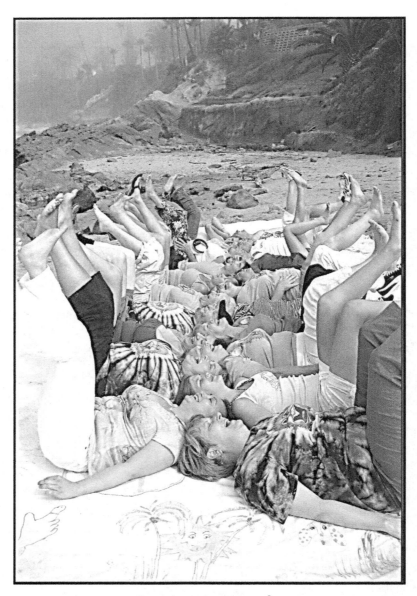

Centipede

Lie on the back, the first person with their head to the center and their feet to the right, the next person with their head to the center but their feet to the left. (Your head is close to that of the next person, while their body extends away in the direction opposite your own body.) Make a line. Kick legs, shake arms, etc.   6 – 10

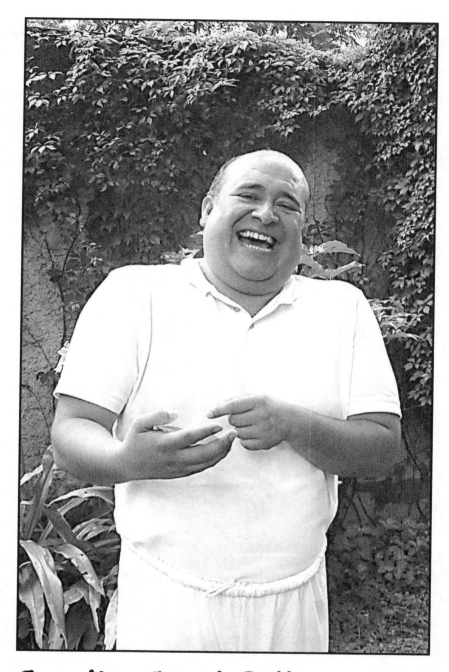

Credit Card Bill (Visa Bill)

In the hands hold an imaginary bill; open the hands
(palms towards you), laugh at what you see; show your
palms and share with others.   3 – 6

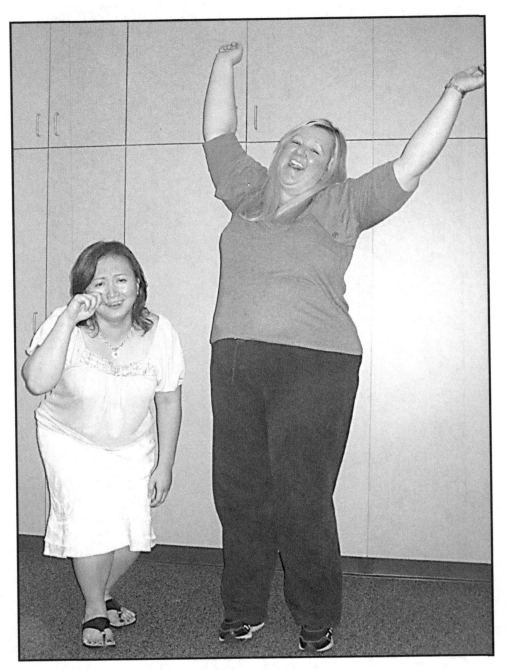

Crying

Cry while sliding down to a crouch; then happily laugh your way up. Repeat several times.   4 – 6 [Omitted 2015]

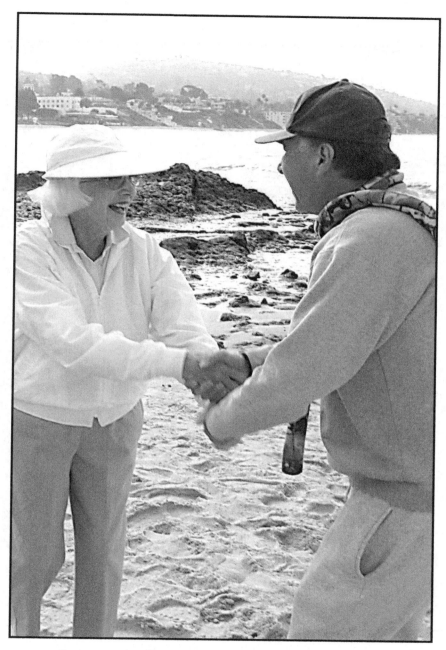

Double Handshake

One person crosses hands, shakes two hands at a time
with the other. Move around and perform with many.
Can jump up and down; sway arms in and out, side to
side, etc. 3 – 7

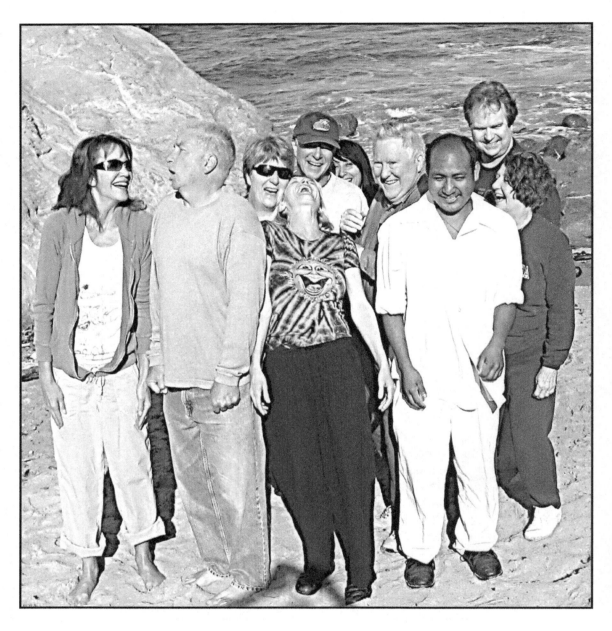

Elevator

Stand close together in a group, laughing nervously as
the elevator jiggles, doors open and close, bouncing
around. Then doors open and everyone bursts out! 3 - 6

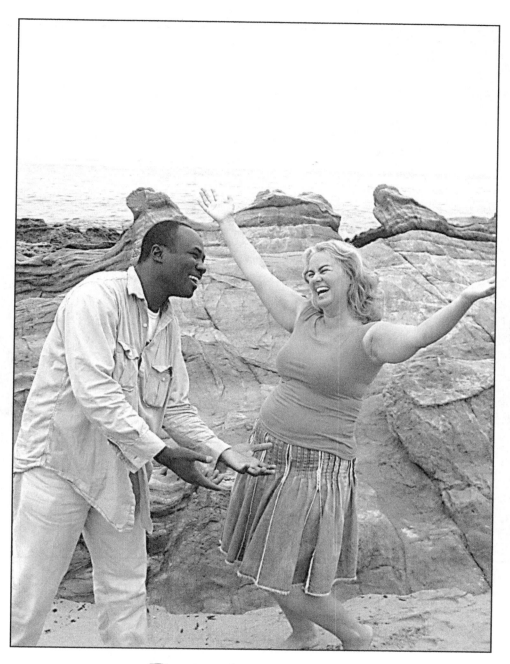

Forgiveness

Offer forgiveness, arms apart and palms open; apologize and ask forgiveness of others. Forgive yourself, forgive everyone. (Alternate with "Argument" p. 14) 2 – 5

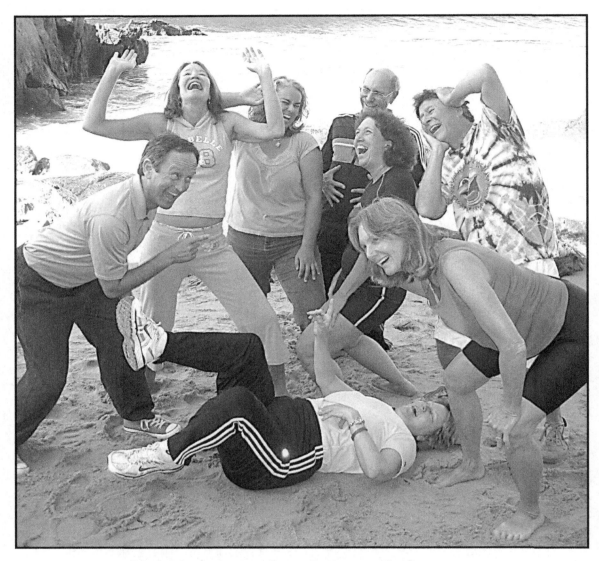

Gibberish Punchlines
(Gibberish Joke)

One person pretends to tell (in gibberish) the last few words of a "joke". When they finish, all laugh as though it was the funniest thing they'd ever heard. (From Laguna Laughter Club. This is not one of Dr. Kataria's Foundation Exercises; we just love it so much, we *had* to include it.) 2 - 10

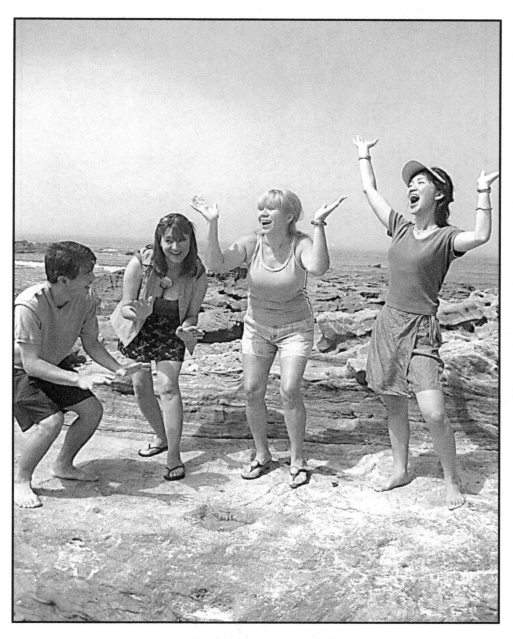

Gradient

Start with a smile, let it grow to a gentle giggle; allow to slowly build, in vigor and volume, until everyone is roaring. Let it diminish back to gentle. 4 – 10

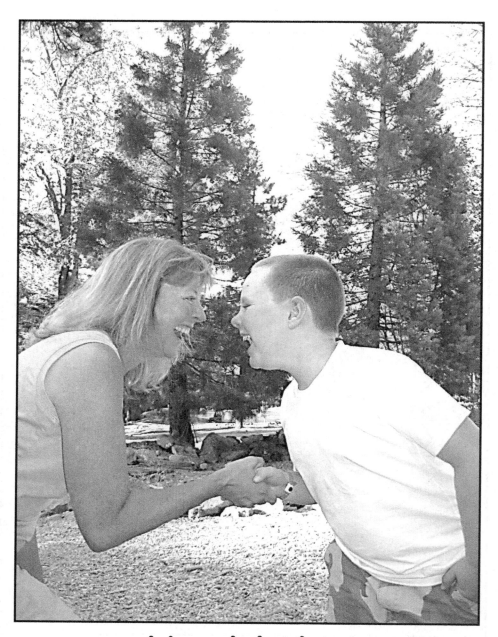

Handshake
(Western Greeting)

Shake another person's hand and laugh, warmly or robustly.   3 – 6

28

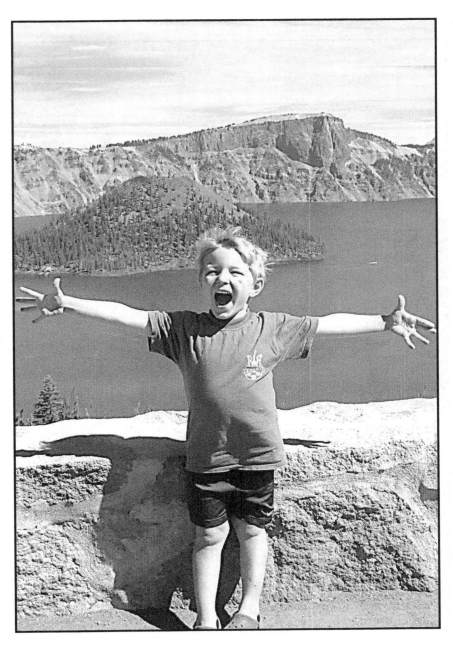

Hearty

Spread your arms up to the sky, tilt your head back and let out a big laugh which shakes your whole heart. Can bounce, or jump up and down (doing so is good for the lymphatic system). 4 – 9

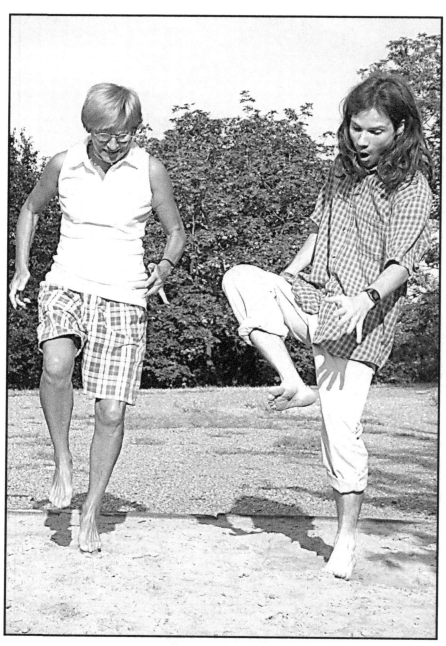

Hot Sand

Walking on very hot sand. "Yeow!- ha-ha-ha-ha!" Move around, wipe hand towards feet, blow to cool the feet with the breath, etc. 6 – 9 [Omitted 2015]

30

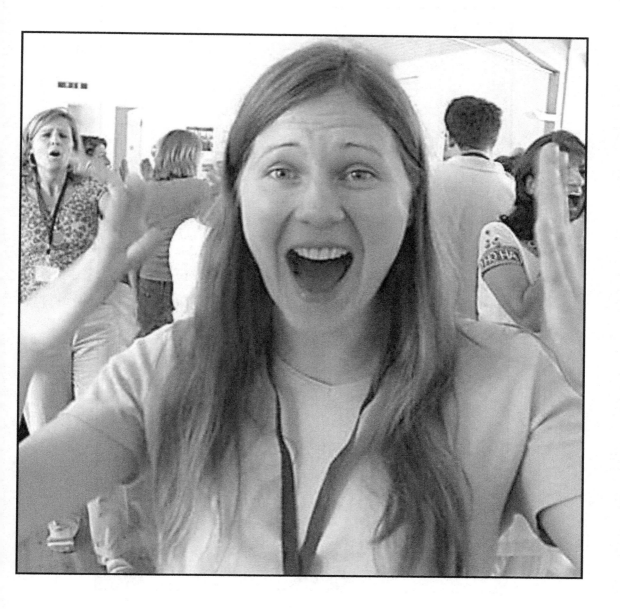

Hot Soup

Stick out tongue, shake hands up and down at wrists as if you have just had very spicy soup; hands wave heat off the tongue. Can help others blow the heat off their tongues. 3 – 6

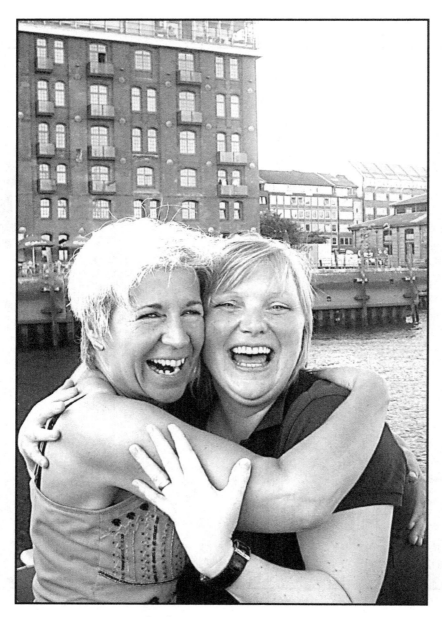

Hugging
(Heart to Heart,
Intimacy Laughter)

Laugh as you gently hug one another; feel each other's laughter.   2 – 4   [Omitted 2015]

32

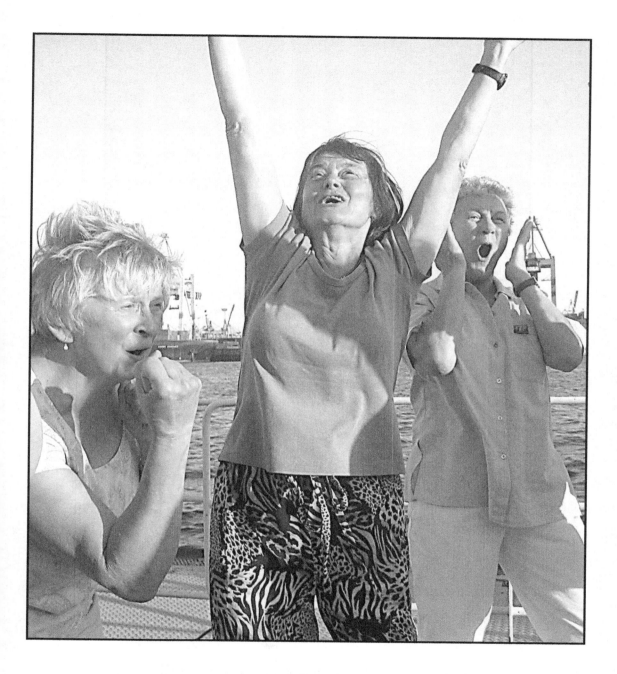

Jackpot

Pull out the winning lottery ticket, raise arms in celebration: "We're rich!"   5 – 10

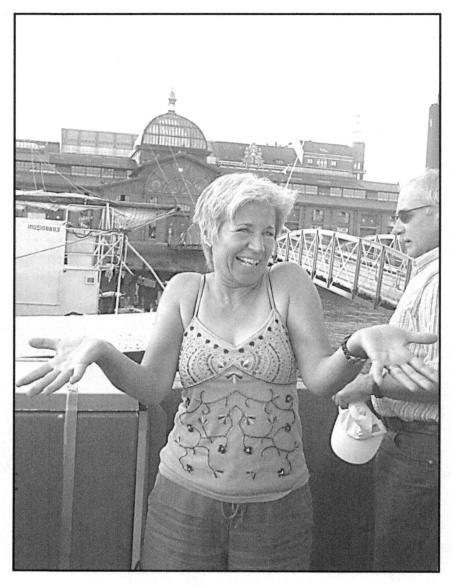

Just Laughing
(Laughing for No Reason)

A passerby has just asked "Why are you all laughing?"
Palms up, elbows bent, shoulders shrug: "We're just...
laughing, for no reason!" 2 – 5

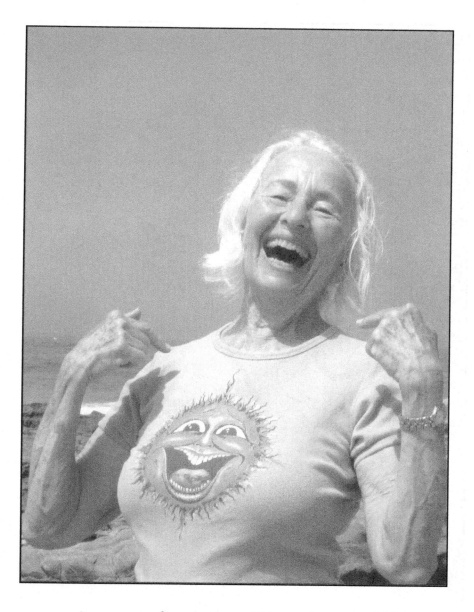

Laugh at Yourself

Point finger at your heart area (may use both hands) with a small movement. "I take myself *so* seriously sometimes – ha ha ha!", "It's okay to laugh at myself, I don't need to be perfect." Can point to head, belly, other body parts. 1 – 3

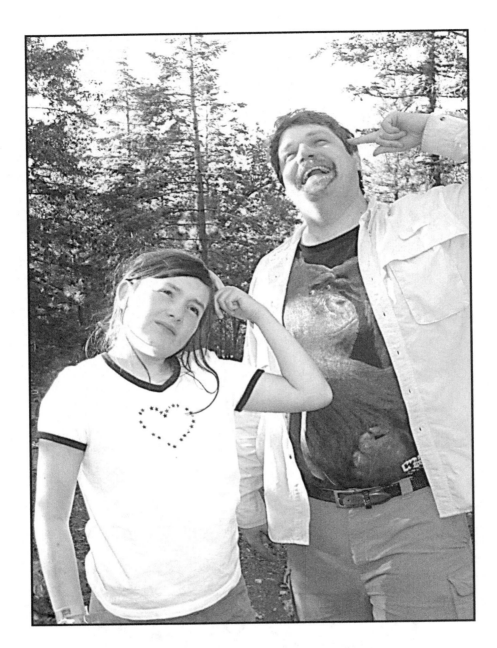

Laughter Center

Point finger to head; seek, then find, and point to others'/ your brain's "Laughter Center" (could be anywhere: temple, crown, occipital ridge in back). Repeat, finding the Laughter Center in other locations. 1 – 3

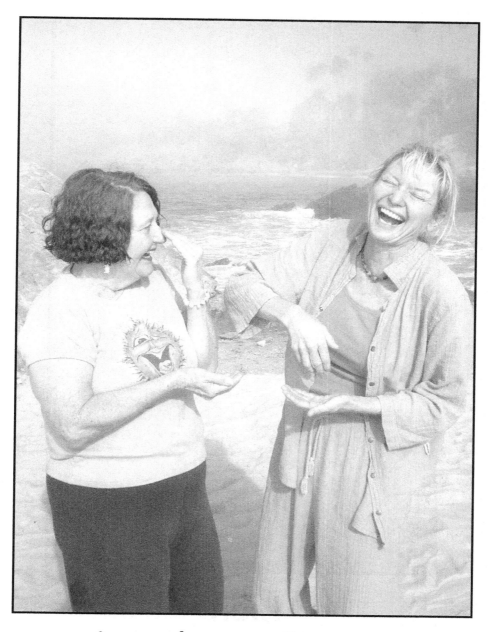

Laughter Cream
(Laughter Lotion)

Squeeze tube into hand (or scoop out of a jar), then apply (to self, and to others). Where you place it, it makes that part jiggle and laugh. 2 – 5

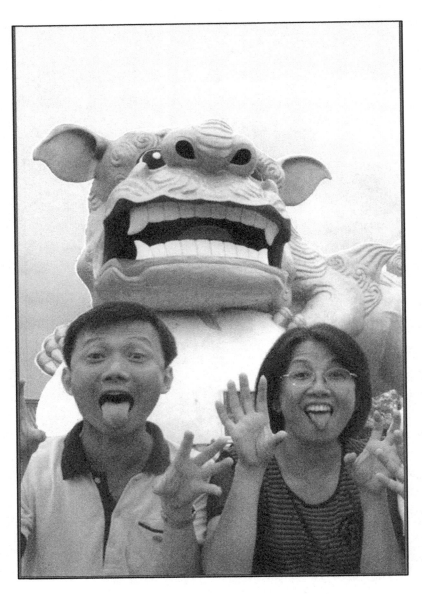

Lion

Stick tongue way out and down towards the chin; big smile; eyebrows lift high, eyes open wide; hands to the sides of the face shaped like a lion's paws (fingers up, thumbs to sides); roar laughter deep from the belly. Can also be "frightened" by the other lions. Then, pounce back! 2 – 6

38

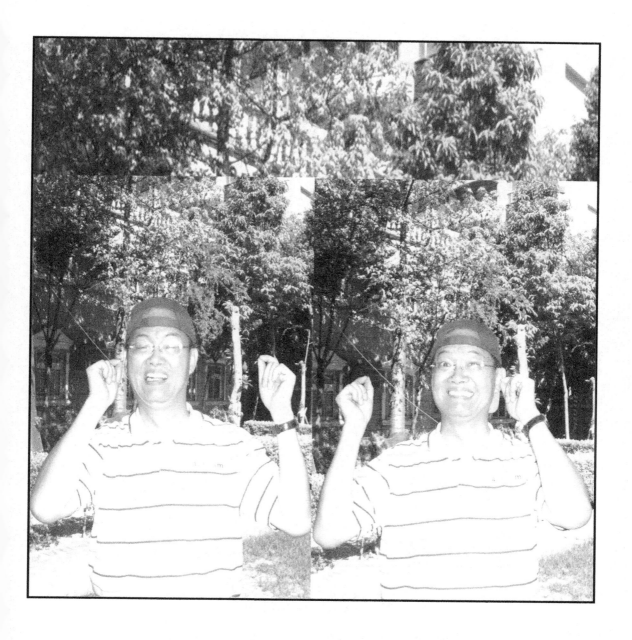

Mental Floss

Wrap floss around hands; "clean out" the brain, tongue, between and around any and all body parts.   2 – 5

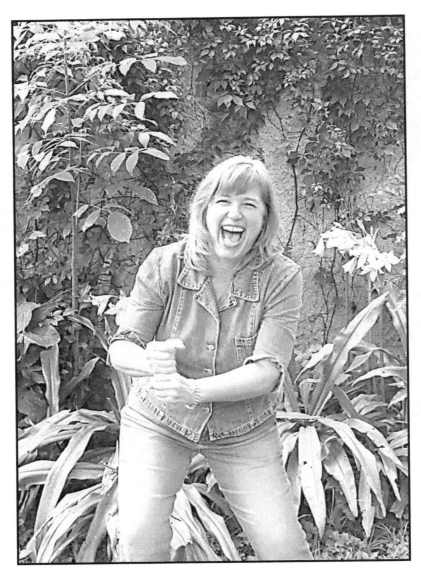

Milk Curd

(Churning Butter, Tak-Choum)

There's a churning-stick in a barrel; lift the stick up and down, or in back-and-forth movements (as if a rope was attached), with repetitive laugh-sounds (as in "Tak-Choom" sounds).   6 – 10   [Omitted 2015]

40

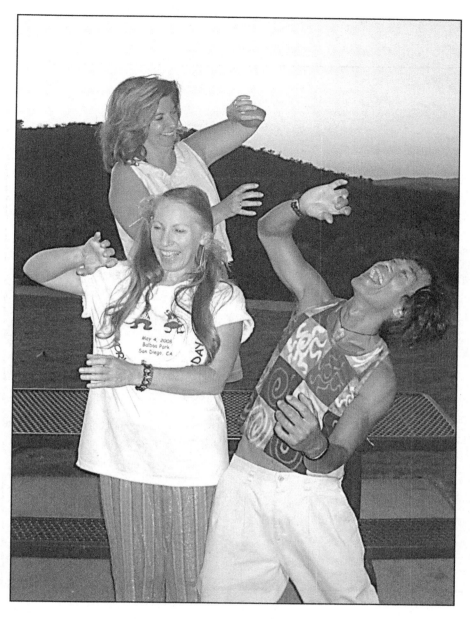

Milkshake (Lassi)

Hold two imaginary glasses of milk. Pour one into the other, saying "Aee..." Pour the second into the first, saying (a little higher) "Aeee…" Then lean back, "drink" and howl. Look around and nod at the others, what a great milkshake you have – and so do they! 4 – 8

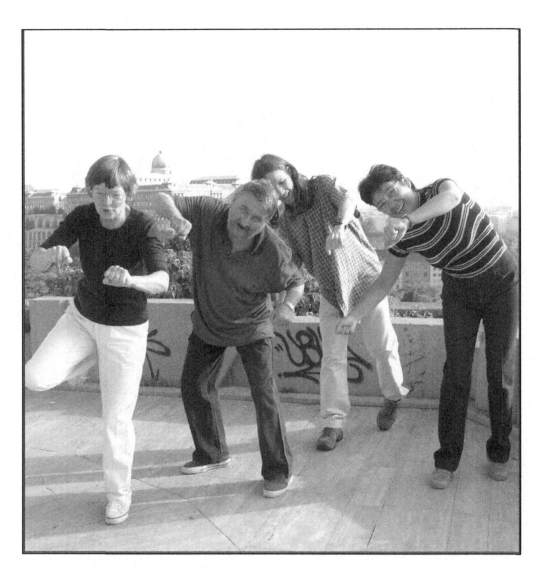

Motorbike (Motorcycle)

It takes three times to start the engine (turning the handle and pushing down one leg). First: "*Ha*-ha-ha-ha-ha." Second: "*HA*-ha-ha-ha-ha-ha." Then it starts: "Ha-ha-ha-ha-ha…" Drive all around on your laugh-powered bike. (Similar: "Motorboat", "Lawnmower") 6 – 10

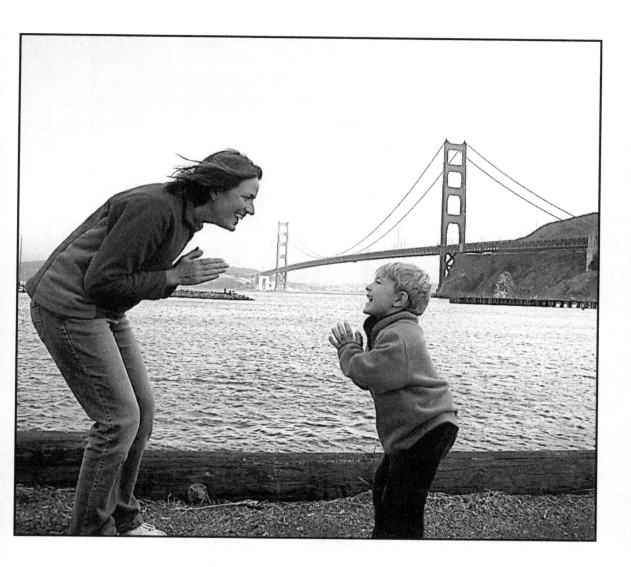

Namaste
(Indian Greeting)

Palms of the hands together in front of your heart. Bow slightly, keeping eye contact. See and laugh with their Child Within, behind the physical eyes. 1 – 3

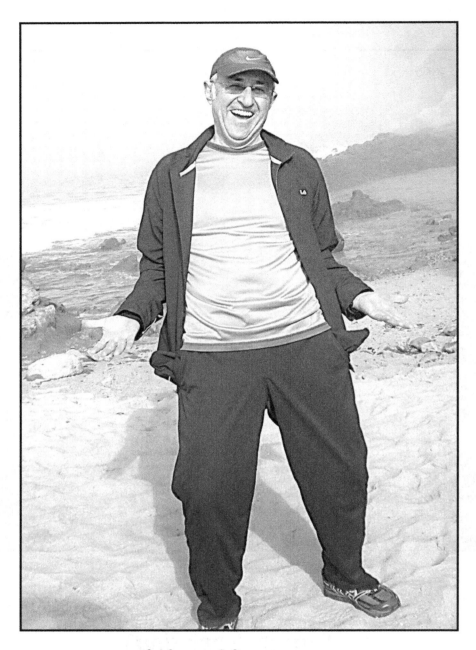

No Money
(Empty Pockets)

Show empty pockets, laugh with palms up. It doesn't really matter! (Follow with "Jackpot" p. 33) 1 – 4

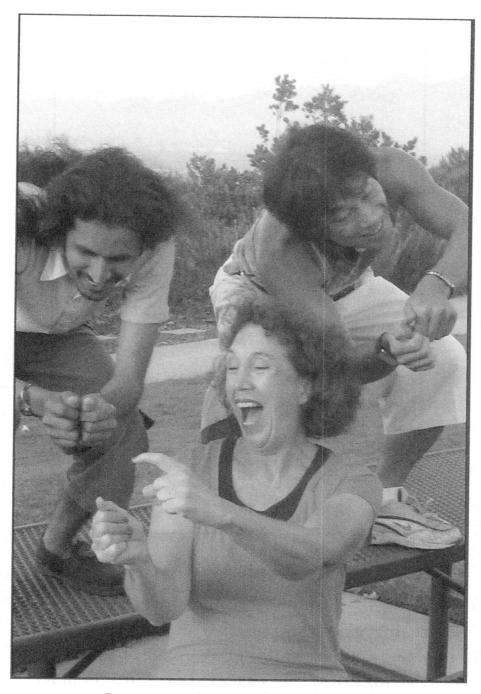

One Centimeter

Measure just from thumb tip to thumb joint; it's over so fast! (Precede with "One Meter" p. 46) 1 – 4

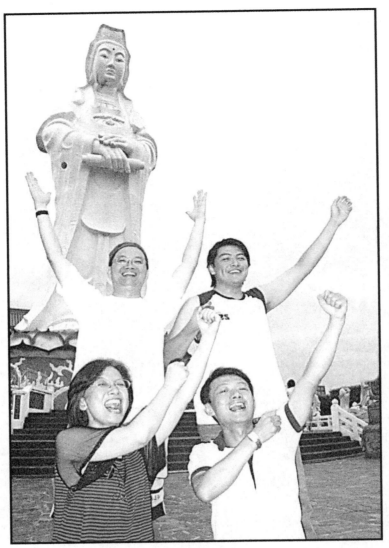

One Meter

As if measuring a length of cloth, start with arms up to
one side, the hands close together. Move one arm along
front of body, as if measuring: 1) To the other arm's
elbow, saying "Aee." 2) To that same arm's shoulder
joint, saying (a little higher) "Aee;" then 3) To the other
shoulder joint and then arms wide apart, head slightly
back; celebrate having succeeded in measuring a meter.
Look around at the others – they've succeeded, too! 3 – 8

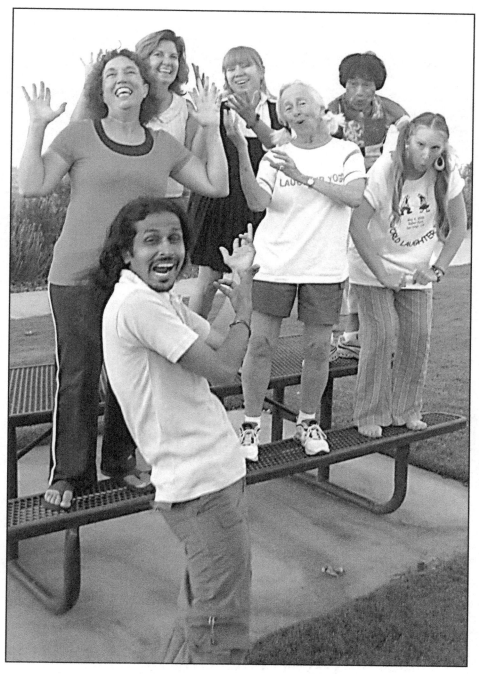

Orchestra Laughter

People group into (laughter-) instrument sections;
conductor directs which group(s) laugh, and when. 5 – 9
[Omitted 2015]

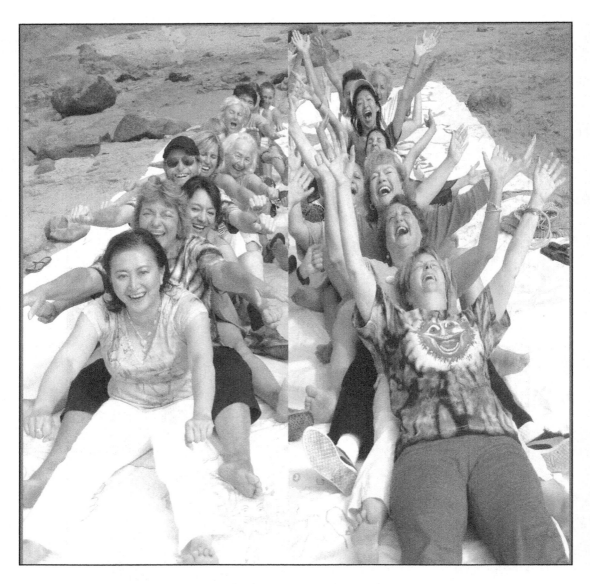

Rowing
(Row the Boat)

Sit with the legs straddling another person, arms in front.
Pretend you are rowing, "Aeee; aeee..."; after two to
four times, lean back and howl, your head resting on the
belly of the person behind. 7 - 10

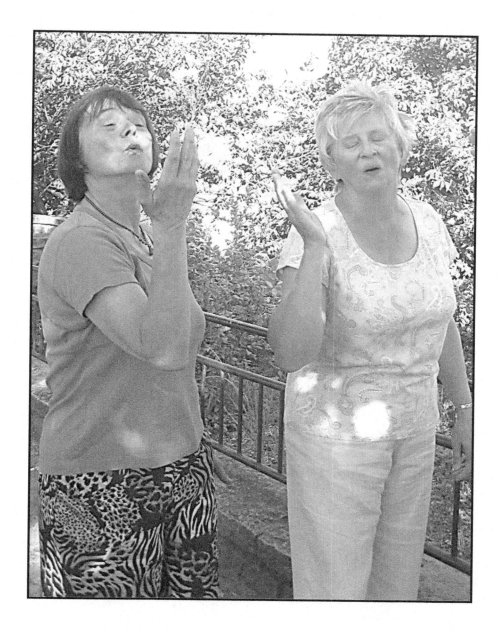

Royal

Hand gently open, wave like the Queen of England
(rotating arm at elbow joint). Can blow kisses, lift the
pinky finger delicately. Enjoy the praise of the adoring
crowds. 1 – 2 [Omitted 2015]

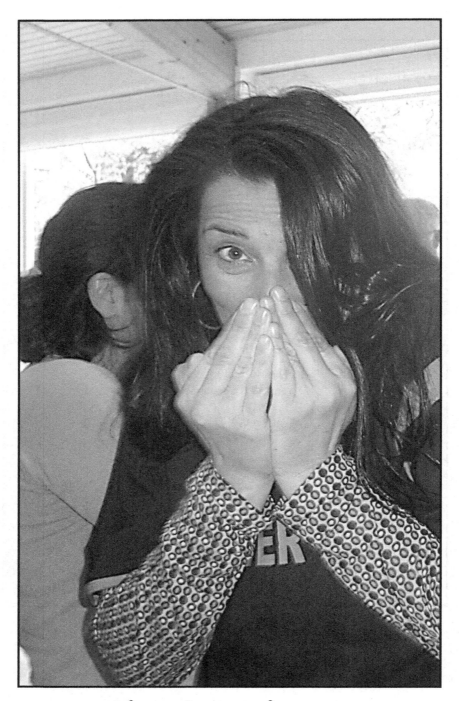

Shy Laughter

Hands in front of face, giggling; peek out sometimes and laugh; then cover the face again.   1 – 3

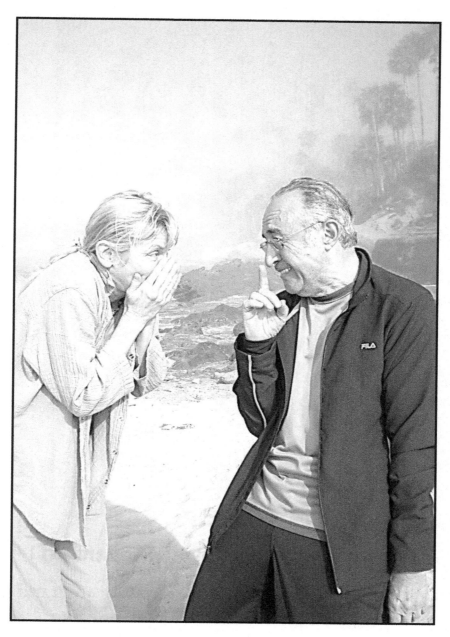

Silent

As if someone is sleeping nearby, laugh very quietly (so as to not wake them up). Can "Shush!" each other. (Good to follow with an outwardly expressive exercise like "Hearty Laughter" p. 29) 1 – 4

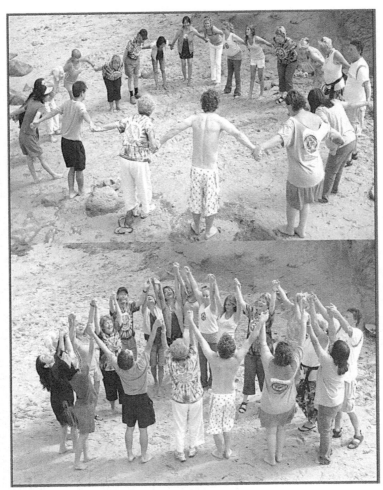

Vowels
(Touch the Sky, Vowel Movement)

Form a wide circle holding hands. Step forward, raising hands, saying each vowel sound and bursting into laughter. After each letter-laugh, step back to the starting position. "A (ay);" then "E (ee);" "I (aye);" "O (oh);" "U (yoo);" and "Y (why)." Can also be performed without holding hands: start with the arms down by the sides; raise the arms above the head as you come forward. Can use the vowel sounds of several languages. 7 – 10

BREATHING EXERCISES

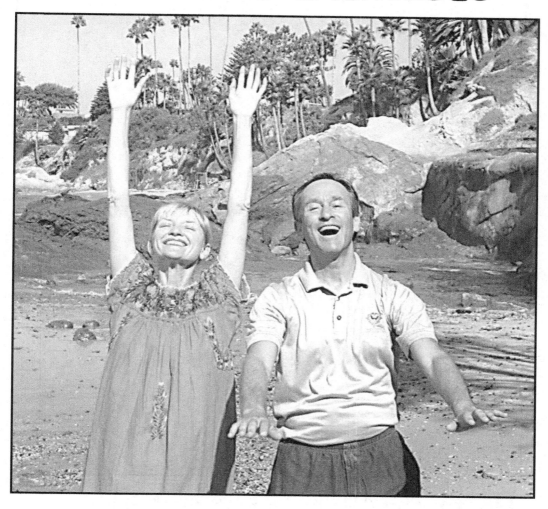

Arms Up the Front Deeply inhale while bringing the two arms up above the head (palms face forward). Exhale fully while lowering arms.

To make a Laughter Exercise: On the exhalation, laugh while lowering the arms. Can walk around, continue laughing as you raise the arms again and then lower/raise at will. 1 – 4

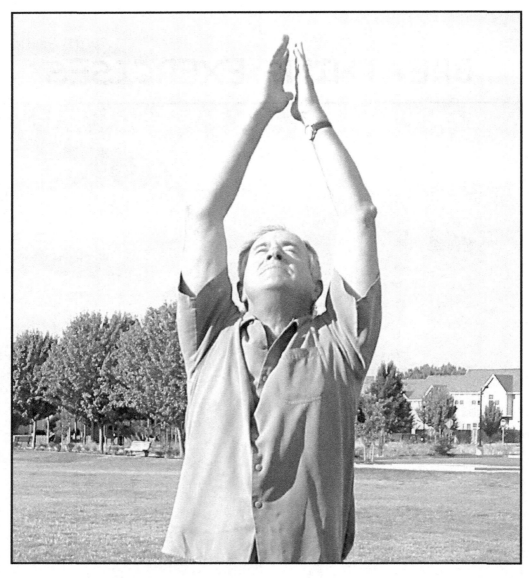

Hastasana ("Ha-ha-ha-hastasana", Palms Together Above Head) To prepare, bring palms together above the head with arms straight. Inhale fully, and exhale completely (keeping the arms up).

As a Laughter Exercise: While exhaling, walk around (arms remaining above the head with palms together) as you nod, smile and laugh, making eye contact with others. 1 – 4

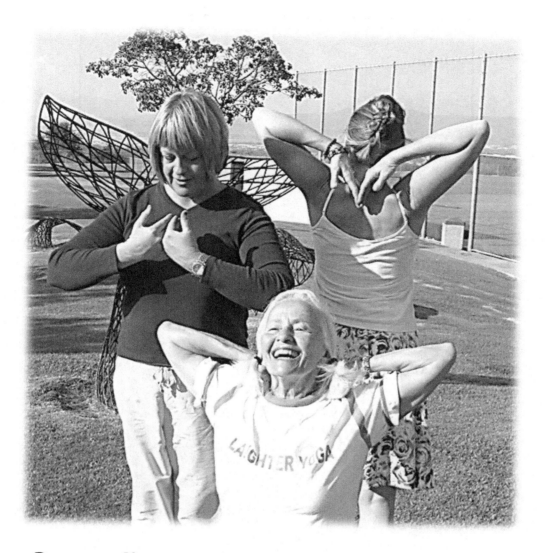

Butterfly Wings (Reverse Prayer,
"Montalbanasana") Place backs of fingers together,
then bring arms up and behind head (hands reach for the
level of the shoulder blades). Inhale fully, stretching
elbows wide apart. Keep the arms where they are as you
exhale completely.

As a Laughter Exercise: On the exhale, walk around
(arms up and behind the head); laugh, nod, and smile
while connecting with others. 2 – 5

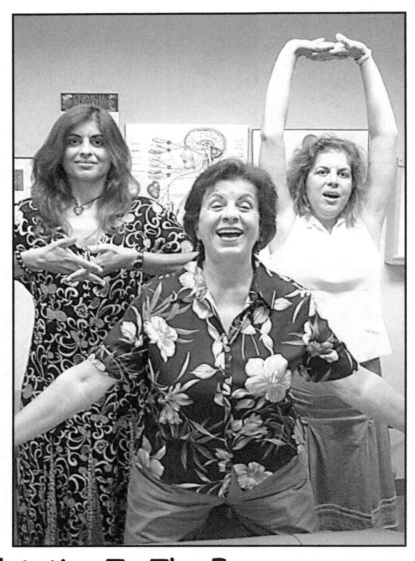

Salutation To The Fun

Salutation To The Fun Interlace fingers below the waist, palms towards belly. Inhaling, bring hands to face, then reverse so palms are towards the sky, extending arms. Exhaling, separate fingers and lower arms down by sides of thighs.

To add Laughter: Stretch the arms up and hold; when you can't hold the breath any longer, burst out laughing. Can move around, interact; return arms up and lower as desired. 2 - 6

OTHER EXERCISES (from Dr. Kataria's foundation practices)

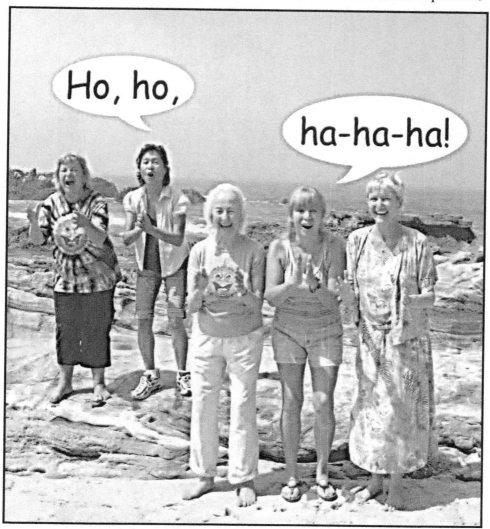

"Ho, ho, ha-ha-ha!" Everyone does simultaneously: Clap hands together in Cha-Cha rhythm ("One, Two, One-Two-Three") making the sounds "Ho, ho, ha-ha-ha!" Walk around, smiling and making good eye contact. (Perform frequently, to conclude the practice of a laughter exercise, and to ground the happy body chemistry with an easily accessible physical "anchor".) 3 - 9

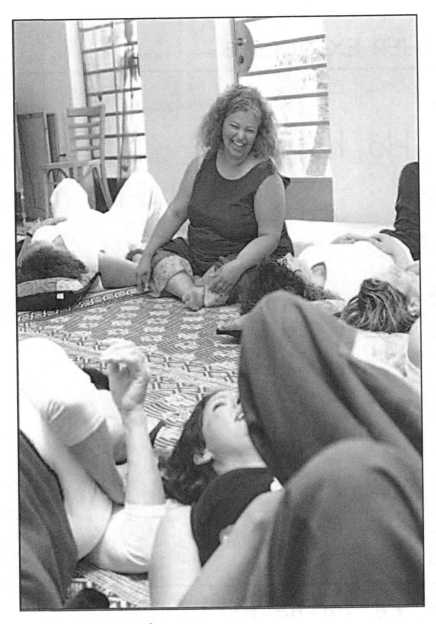

Laughter Meditation Version 1: Sit with eyes open. (Version 2: Lie on the floor with eyes closed.) Allow laughter to rise up spontaneously, any way that feels good. (Often performed for three to ten minutes as the final Laughter Exercise before Relaxation.) 1 – 10

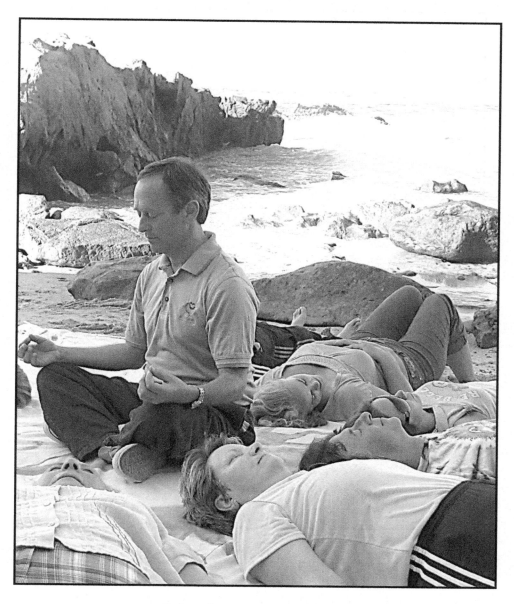

Relaxation

Lie down, or sit comfortably, with the back straight.
Leader guides participants to relax every body part.
(Always end a laughter session with a period of
relaxation to integrate the health benefits.)   0 – 1

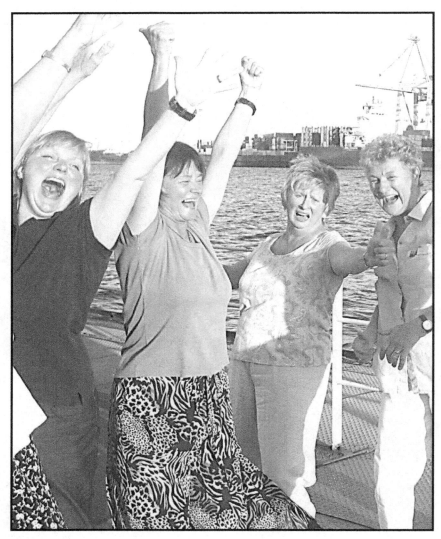

"Very good, very good, Yay!"

Everyone does simultaneously. Clap hands together once (saying "Very good"), clap together again ("Very good"); then separate arms wide apart with thumbs up (or fingers wide apart) saying "Yay!" Repeat three or more - can be *many* more - times. (Perform frequently to conclude the practice of a laughter exercise, as well as to encourage a sense of childlike playfulness.) 3 – 10

Aloha Laughter Inhaling, raise both arms up; say "Alo-o-o-" for a long breath; at the very end of the breath, come down with a firm "Ha-a-a!" and continue to laugh deeply. 3 - 8

Creative Laughter One at a time, each person does spontaneous and playful: 1. Sounds, 2. Faces/Grimaces, and 3. Actions/Gestures, for 10 or more seconds; the others observe and react playfully. 2 – 6 [Omitted 2015]

   Variation: Creative Laughter - Pass It Around One person pretends to have an invisible object (a piece of rope, a lump of clay) which can be stretched or molded into *anything*. It can pass through their body, be heavy as lead or light as air - "It" can have any shape, any properties. They play with this invisible stuff for 5-10 seconds while the others admire and laugh. Then they pass It to another person, who plays with and changes It. Continue passing It around, everyone having a chance to transform and play with It. 3 - 9

   Variation: Follow the Leader Each person does any movement/laughter exercise for three to ten seconds, the others copying them at the same time. 4 - 8

Electric Shock Reach out a hand as if to shake hands; an electrostatic shock comes from the other person's hand. Fun surprise! 3 - 6

Household Chores Wash dishes; pass the vacuum cleaner; clean windows; fold laundry… 4 - 8

Laughter Revival (A Laughter Scene) A group of laughers finds an unconscious person. In gibberish they argue for a few moments about calling emergency help. One person suggests (in gibberish): "All we need to do is share laughter energy." All place their hands over the person, waving and laughing; the "unconscious" person slowly regains consciousness. Celebrate and continue on together. 3 - 9

Party Laughter
Use several previous exercises: Meet the partygoers (Greeting/Handshake and Namaste); "Oops, I left something at home" (Cellphone Laughter); Ate Spicy Food (Hot Soup Laughter). Make groups of twos and threes and laugh over imaginary drinks. Have "very amusing" joke-filled conversations (entirely in gibberish). 3 - 7

+ Added by Dr. Kataria in 2015 +
(When Dr. Kataria published a revised set of Foundation Exercises in 2015, the following were omitted: American Cowboy, Calcutta, Crying, Royal, Hot Sand, Hugging, Milk Curd, Orchestra, Creative.)

Aches and Pains
Point to, or place hands on, an area where you've ever felt an ache or pain (foot, knee, back, neck, head, teeth, etc.). "Boo hoo" a moment, then laugh aloud. Continue, indicating several other areas (sympathizing with others). 1 – 6

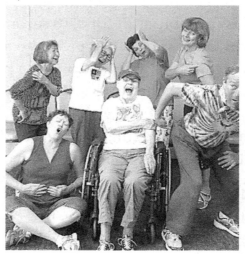

Airplane Variation:
Airport: 1. Pretend you're late and run around with bags. 2. Get a boarding card. 3. Wave 'Goodbye' to your bags disappearing on the conveyor belt. 4. Get into the airplane.

Bird Variation: Chicken Laughter
Place hands by sides (or on shoulders) with elbows jutting out; flap around and squawk/laugh like a chicken. 3 - 5

Guru Laughter Put one hand atop your head: "I learn from my mistakes". Put the other hand atop the first: "I learn from others' mistakes". Walk around with both hands on the head, nodding and laughing, acknowledging that we all make mistakes and learn therefrom. 2 - 5

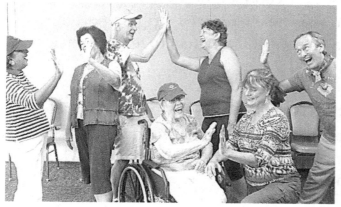

High Five

Raise one arm with palm facing away; slap another's hand: "We did it, we won!" "Give me five!" 4 – 8

Magic Laughter Extend the arms in front, hands as fists. Raise the pointer fingers of both hands. Tap the inside edge of the hands together, saying "Ay" (pronounced as in "day"). Separate them, then bring together again with "Ay". The third time, raise two fingers (the pointer and middle fingers) up on each hand, as if you've made them magically multiply. "Ha haaa – I did magic!" 3 - 5

Milkshake Variations

a) After combining the two cups, you begin to drink; it tastes funny, so : 1.) pour the milkshake out over your head and behind your back; &/or : 2.) pour it out on the earth in front of you.

b) Share the milkshake with others by pouring it down the back of their shirt, tossing above their head, etc. 2 - 10

Sports Theme
Pretend to be participating in any desired sport: Juggling, Basketball, Baseball, Football, Volleyball, Sumo Wrestling, Weightlifting, Javelin Throwing, Soccer, etc.

Exaggerate the moves with deep breaths, turning to laughter. 3 - 10

Waxing Laughter Pretending to place wax on the arms, move one palm over the other arm from elbow to wrist. One application with "Ay"; a second application, "Ay…" The third time, pull from wrist to elbow, as if stripping off the wax, yell "Ah- ha ha ha ha!" It feels great to tear that hair out with laughter! 2 - 6

Wi-Fi Laughter Have the hands by the upper sides of the head. Make fists but with the pointer finger extended. Walk around, seeking a Wi-Fi network connection… when you find one, "Ha ha!" 1 – 3

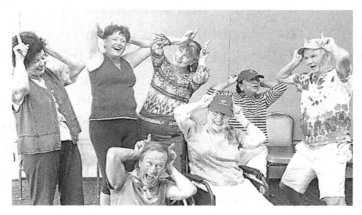

Zoo Animal Theme Each person walks around acting like any animal they choose (Elephant, Lion, Kangaroo, Monkey, Snake, Chicken, Penguin, Duck…). Can change to another animal whenever desired. 2 – 9

- END of Part 1 "Foundation Exercises" -

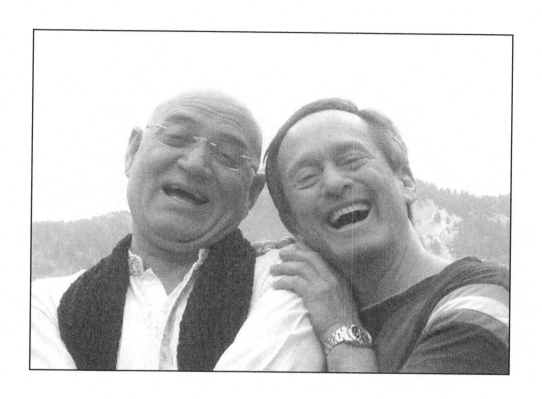

Laughter Buddies
Madan Kataria and Jeffrey Briar

Wilderswil, Switzerland

May 2011

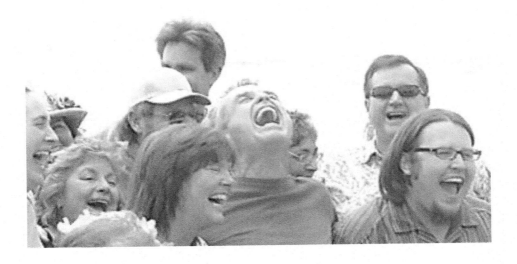

Dr. Kataria's Foundation Laughter Exercises

Please visit
The Laughter Yoga Institute www.LYInstitute.org
Laughter Yoga International www.laughteryoga.org

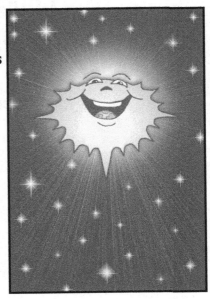

Part 2

Encyclopedia of Laughter Exercises

Compiled, written and edited by Jeffrey Briar

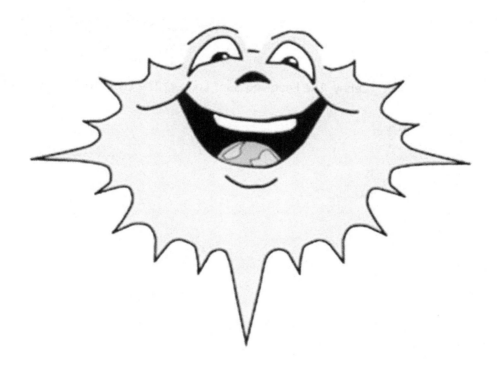

450 Laughter Practices
for Health, Fun and Friendship

From The Laughter Yoga Institute

www.LYInstitute.org

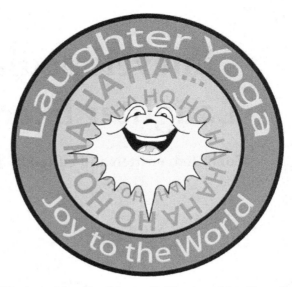

Encyclopedia of Laughter Exercises (black-and-white version)
(Section Two of *Laughter Exercises: The Great Big Anthology*)

Encyclopedia of Laughter Exercises

Compiled, written &/or edited by Jeffrey Briar

All exercises are performed *while laughing.* No real words are spoken, except by the Leader while giving instructions. All word examples given below are presented to indicate the feeling being expressed, but participants do not actually speak in any real language. They only make laughter sounds, or speak in gibberish.

Accountant Laughter: (See "CPA Laughter".)

Age Laughter: Laugh in the style you would sound when you are double your current age; half of your current age; 10 years older; or 20; or 30 years older; 10 years younger; as a child; as a newborn baby.

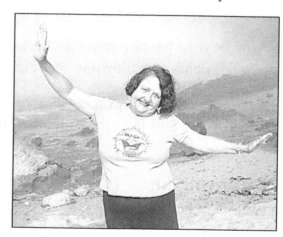

Airplane Laughter: Spread the arms wide. Take off, fly around, buzz each other; fly into a storm; land, discharge passengers.

Aloha Laughter: (Kataria style):
Raise arms high above head, saying "Alo - o-o -o-o"; when near the end of the breath, bend forward at the waist saying "Ha –ha-ha-ha-ha!" Continue laughing deeply. (Option: slap the thighs, and dash around making eye contact with others.)

Aloha Laughter (Wilson style): Arms wave and hips sway side to side like a Hawaiian Dancer, saying "Alo-ha-ha-ha-ha!" Walk around and wave, shake hands with and greet each other.

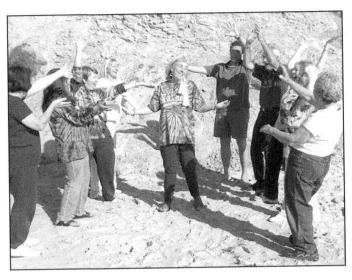

Angel Wash: Form two lines. Person at the end walks down the center between the two lines; the others applaud and cheer, expressing gratitude for the angelic being in front of them. Each person follows, so everyone gets a chance to be both the "angel walking down" and someone in the line of supportive cheerers.

Ants in your Pants Laughter: Run around wiping ants off your (and others') pants, jumping and leaping as though being nipped terribly.

Autumn Leaves Laughter: Cling to a tree, a breeze comes; one by one we drop off, and float in the wind. Then bunch up together, and: "All Fall Down!"

Award Night: One person is receiving an award, expressing gratitude, surprise, relief, humility, pride, etc. The others are applauding their friend at

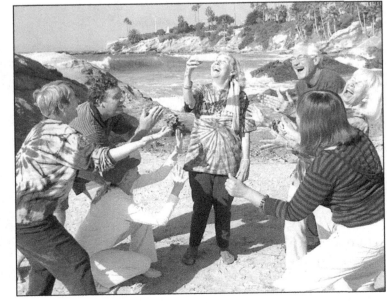

the joyful surprise: "Hooray, you won!" Let several people be the Award Recipient.

Babbling Brook Laughter: Act like a little river, making burbly bubbly small fast laughs and moving fluidly with small flickery motions.

Bad Babysitter Laughter: Watch TV; smoke; put booze in the baby's bottle; have friends/boyfriends over; talk incessantly on the phone. (Pair with "Good Babysitter".)

Bad Date 1: Be a woman, on a date, in tight clothes – then your blouse tears and everything falls out.

Bad Date 2: Be a man, on a date, in tight clothes – then your pants rip…

Balloon Laughter 1: Blow up a pretend balloon with laughter and then let it out fast, your body squiggling and fluttering around like a balloon deflating.

Balloon Laughter 2: Blow up the balloon; bigger, bigger… it pops, and everyone laughs in relief.

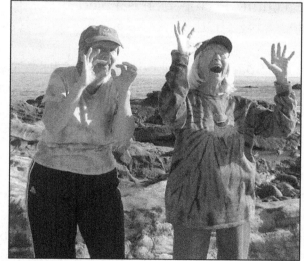

Balloon-Popping Laughter: Try to pop each other's imaginary balloons, which can be attached to your ankles, wrists, chests, bottoms, noses...

Banana Peel Laughter: (See "Peel a Banana".)

Band (Marching Band): In a circle. Each person plays a musical instrument (trumpet, violin, trombone, harp, drums, etc.) making laughter sounds; the others copy (like "Follow the Leader"). Go around so each person can "play." After everyone has had a turn, strut around like a marching band, but all disorganized. Can play any instrument from those done previously, or a new one; change to another instrument whenever you wish.

Baseball Laughter, 1: Ready to catch a high fly ball --- here it comes, here it comes --- you catch it, and save the game!
    Baseball Laughter, 2: The fly ball comes to you; you drop it – "Oh well, it's only a game!"
    Baseball Laughter, 3: With a Partner. Pitcher pitches, Batter swings - whatever happens, we just laugh. (Batter can miss the ball, hit it with his head, grab the ball in his teeth… Pitcher can catch it between her knees, have the ball pass right through her, the ball goes overhead and gets caught by an outfielder, etc.)

Be a Quilt: Each person is a piece. We stitch each other together and make a big quilt. Then we admire ourselves.

Be the Sparkles: Embody the sparkles of sunlight on the ocean (or lake)'s surface. Imagine the sparkles infuse you: be a laughing "Being of Light".
    Variation: Be the sparkles on the waves as they break.

Beach Surprise: Lying on the beach, you are startled by sand falling; or an ice cream cone being dropped, or water splashing on you.

Becoming a Were-Animal Laughter: As if being bewitched by a magic spell, slowly turn into: a puppy dog; a pussycat; a bunny rabbit; a majestic eagle; a frantic monkey; a lumbering hippopotamus; a massive whale, etc.

Becoming a Werewolf Laughter: The moon rises. You see it and realize what's coming... Gradually turn into a snarling fun-werewolf.

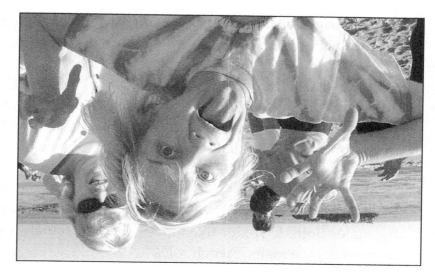

Bee Chase: Being chased by a bee or bees. (When you are stung, it *tickles*, it doesn't sting.) **Variation: Friendlies Bee Chase:** Being chased by a swarm of friendly bees ("Oh, you guys!...").

Bee Stings Your Tongue Laughter: Your tongue swells up, you can speak only in round-mouthed gibberish.

Being Born: Be a baby, crammed inside the womb. Then come forth, and celebrate and delight in every single thing that comes to your awareness: sunlight, wind, your own breath, your fingerprints, other people – *every single* thing! Everything is amazing.

      Variation: In groups. One (or several) people are those being born. The others are birth attendants, friends and family, who applaud and rejoice, welcoming the newly-arriving babies being born. Reverse roles.

Belly Button Laughter: "I'll show you *yours*, if *you'll* show me *mine*!" Just point and celebrate - no need to actually lift up your shirt.

Bemused Laughter: Lips are closed, cheeks with a goodly smile; eyes open just a little, as if you are remembering a mildly amusing incident. Share winks and knowing looks with one another.

Bird Menagerie Laughter: Make laughter-sounds like different birds: seagull (high pitch), crow (caw), songbird, duck, rooster, etc.

Birthing: Act like you are delivering a baby. It could be very easy: a little squat, and out it pops! Or with struggle – but always laughing. Then show off/share babies with each other. Can swap babies, juggle them, throw like a football, tickle them, try to put a bottle in their mouth, etc. (Also see "Die Laughing" sequence.)

Black Widow Laughter: With a partner. One is the female, the other the male. Both do spider-like moves; then the female bites and "eats" (consumes) the male. Switch roles.

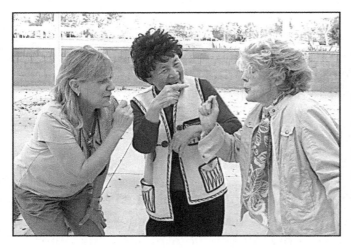

Blowing Bubbles Laughter: Pretend to blow (and gleefully pop) your and others' soap bubbles.

Blue Danube Waltz (in Gibberish): One person is the "conductor," others in three groups. Conductor points to the others to do the famous waltz. ...the 'ha', the 'hee' & the 'ho' sections, alternate the parts. (Works well with 12 or more people.)

Boo hoo, ha ha: Cry a little, laugh a little. Go back and forth. (Similar to "Crying Laughter," but can alternate as quickly or slowly as you wish.)

Bored Laughter: Act as though bored, with a very easy, almost sarcastic laugh. (Good to follow with "Hearty Laughter".)

74

Boss Quit Today: Everyone just got the news: no more Mister Mean Guy! Celebrate, give high-five, express relief, toss paper clips, etc.

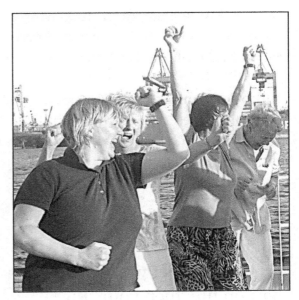

Bowl of Laughter: Hold an imaginary bowl and spoon. Eat your laughter flakes then laugh. Hahahaha, "Less filling, feels great, burns calories!"

Breezing Along with the Breeze: Alone and with others you are a molecule of air, blown by the breeze and wind; low, medium, high; slow, fast, hovering.

Burlesque Dance: Pretend to do a strip-tease dance (stripping off all negativity, self-doubt, sadness, etc.). Make your own "bump and grind" laughter/gibberish-music. Laugh away your cares and doubts; flap your old "negativity-clothes" on the floor, show off your beautiful care-free body, etc.

Bus Stop: In a row. One person resists laughing or smiling; the others try to make them laugh. Switch roles several times.

Butterfly Emerging From Cocoon: Start small in a cocoon; hatch out. Transformed, you spread and dry and admire your wings; and "Now we can fly!"

Butterflies in Your Bathrobe (a variation on "Ants in Your Pants"): You are wearing a bathrobe – filled with butterflies! They are light, tickly sensual, uplifting.   After they tickle you from inside your robe for a few seconds, Let Them Free! Open the robes, release; can do Hearty Laughter in celebration of their freedom.

Buttocks Contraction (pubococcygeus-strengthening; improves bladder control): Uses "Ho, ho, ha-ha-ha" rhythm. Make a fist with each hand for "Ho, ho", contract your buttocks muscles (squeeze butt cheeks together) for "Ha-ha-ha."

Candelabra Laughter: Make yourself into a candelabra. Set your hair on fire, then your hands. Flame on and light each other up.

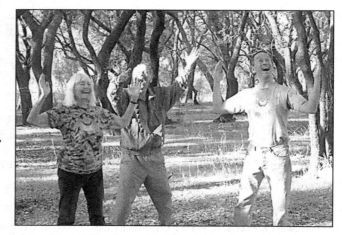

Can't Talk Laughter (Laughing Too Much to Talk): Everyone is laughing so hard that even though you are trying to talk to others, you just can't get any words out. Use body language to indicate you *want* to talk, but you simply cannot; you are cracking up laughing too much. "Sorry, I just – can't – ha ha ha ha hah!" Walk around and interact with many others (all of whom are likewise unable to speak, although trying to do so - but they are laughing too hard).

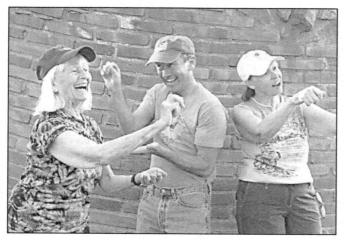

Canvas Painters (Canvas Painting): The world in front of you is a giant canvas. Everyone mime-paints it with "brushes" and "paints" of laughter: use little strokes (hee–hee-hee), big strokes (Ha, ha, ha *ha*!). Squeeze the paint from the tube and use fingers, use a spray can, etc.

Variation: can also playfully paint each other.

Car Won't Start: Make sounds like a car trying, but failing, to start. Turn the key, at first it almost starts, but then it dies away: *Hah* ha ha ha ha…. Try again: *Hah*, ha ha ha ha… After three or four times, it runs: Ha ha ha ha ha ha ha! Drive around and wave at each other.

Changing Diapers: As you are in the middle of changing the baby's diaper, it lets out another soiling. "Hahahahaha" – you just change it again!

Charlie Chaplin Walk:
Turn legs so toes point out. Walk around like Charlie Chaplin; spin a cane, shift head side-to-side, twitch moustache, lift one leg, etc.

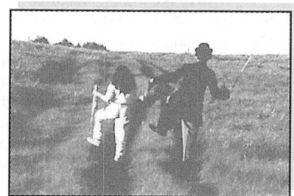

Chasing the Train Laughter: Chase after the train, wave and run – and you catch it! Yay!

Variation: Chase after the train, wave and run – and you *don't* catch it! "No problem – there'll be another train in 5 minutes!"

Chi Massage Laughter: Rub hands together, building up "Laugh Chi". Project to others (can touch hands, or not). Recharge, rubbing hands together again. Send "Laugh Chi" energy forth from the hands: 1) To the earth; 2) To the heavens; 3) To the earth again, etc. 4) To each other; 5) To people who are not present.

Chicken Laughter: Fold arms into wings, lift one leg; dash around, cluck and flap. Stop to peck. Lay an egg.

Christmas-Themed Exercises

Caught Under the Mistletoe Laughter. "Oops! Now we've got to share a kiss…" Just pretend, on the cheek ("I went here on purpose…")

Decorating the Tree: Place globes, garlands, etc. on a tree; gifts below, attach lights, etc. **Variation:** One (or several) people stand in the middle – they "are" the tree. The others decorate them (as above), plug in the electric cord, admire their handiwork.

Gift Opening: Remove an invisible object from its gift wrap with delight – "It's just what I wanted!" Share with others. **Variation**: Everyone opens their gifts at the same time: a gift-opening whirlwind.

Gift – No Biggie Laughter: Waggle finger like in "Naughty-Naughty"; "Maybe I didn't get much, but it was worth it! I don't need a material thing to celebrate and laugh."

Gratitude Goggles: Use fingers to encircle eyes (like 3-D glasses): your vision is transformed! You notice beautiful details of everything and everyone; walk around with joy and thankfulness.

Green Jello Mold: Everyone jiggles and giggles.

Making Small Talk (in Gibberish): Everyone is at a holiday party making small talk with each other, chattering and laughing in gibberish.

Santa Claus: (See "Santa Laughter".)

Shy Gift-giving: Be a 6 year-old; you've made a little card or gift for someone you secretly have a crush on. Milling with eyes averted, trying to be invisible, attempt to sneak your gift into your friend's pocket - sometimes the giggling can't be contained. Can run away; they stop you by catching our eye and laughing because they have a little gift for you in *their* pocket!

Sing traditional songs with laughter words: "Deck the Hall with boughs of holly, 'Ha ha ha ha ha, ha ha, ha, ha!'" "Jingle Bells", "Rudolph the Red-Nosed Reindeer", etc.

Snoring after the Meal: Inhale a snore, exhale laughter.

So-Stuffed Waddle: Meet someone, stick out your tummy and waddle penguin-style towards them. Bump bellies and bounce back laughing.

Variation: Enjoying overindulging together, serving each other second helpings of favorite holiday foods, then getting up from the table and doing the waddle and belly-bump as we take gifts to each other.

Stirring the soup: Everyone pretends they have a big pot of soup in front of them and stirs it with a giant spoon. (See "Making Soup" for photo.)

Too much pumpkin pie laughter (see "Upchuckle").

--- --- --- --- --- --- --- --- --- --- --- --- --- --- --- --- ---

Circus Laughter: Be different characters in the circus: **Trapeze Artist, Lion Tamer, Lion, Tightrope Walker** (see photo, and variations under "Walking a Tightrope"), **Juggler, Elephant, Trained Dogs, Showgirl, Crazy Clowns,** etc.

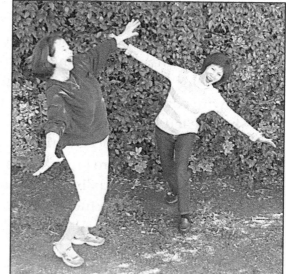

Version 1: Leader declares the "act," everyone does that role. Do three or four different roles (10 to 20 seconds each).

Version 2: Participant's choice: many different acts are happening at the same time. It's a ten-ring circus!

Cloud Laughter: Be big fluffy hovering clouds. Can bump into each other and do "thunderous" laughs. Rain down laughter, giving the world a shower of happiness.

Cocktail Party Laughter: Make groups of two's and three's; laugh with each other over imaginary drinks, gibberish conversations (joke-reacting), spill drinks, apologize. Mix with other groups.

Coming Out of Your Shell: You're a baby bird, folded up inside of an egg. Crack away at the eggshell and burst out, happy to be born. Then fly, joyful and free!

Compassionate Laughter: Sometimes called "Life's Little Stresses", "Free-Floating Hostilities", or "Ha Ha Mantra". An advanced practice because, unlike most of the laughter exercises in this collection, it involves speaking in an actual language.

One person at a time speaks up and shares something which they perceived as an annoyance. For example: "When I was getting ready to leave for this seminar, I couldn't find my car keys." When they finish, following the Leader's cue, everyone gives a gentle, slow laugh: "Ha, ha, ha, ha, ha..." delivered with compassion; a sense of "Oh yeah, I too have forgotten things..." It is best if *every* person can have a chance to share. **Variations:**

"**Small**" - share minor, unimportant things: "Forgot my shoes", "'Got a parking ticket", "Someone cut ahead of me at the market..."

"**Big**" is to share more "charged" things (which are nonetheless met with compassionate "Yeah, me too... Ha, ha, ha, ha, ha..." laughter): "My wife left me for another man", "I declared bankruptcy today", "I was driving, had an accident and my passenger was seriously hurt..."

"**Really Big**" are huge things for which the person speaking couldn't possibly actually be responsible: "Fleas", "The invention of money", "The Spanish Inquisition", all of which are met with compassionate "Oh, yeah, that happens... Ha, ha, ha, ha, ha..."

Constipation Laughter: Squat on an imaginary seat; struggle and strain for a bit… then let it go. What a relief!

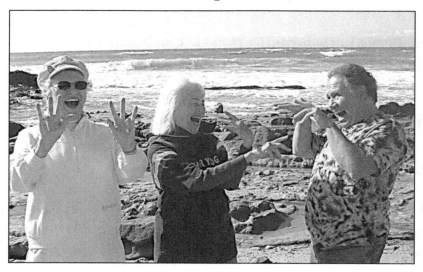

Count Your Blessings: Hold out your hands, fingers open wide. As you bend down the same finger of

80

each hand (both pinkies, both ring fingers, etc.), laugh for three or four seconds while you think of a wonderful blessing in your life: a person, a place, a relationship, an object; something that brings you joy and gratitude. After doing all five fingers, "Share Your Blessings": waggle your blessing-fingers at everyone (and yourself). Follow this with Gradient Laughter or any other hand-related exercise.

CPA Laughter ("Accountant Laughter"): Tap on calculator; talk with phone on shoulder while doing other things with hands. Write things down; put papers into files, put files into filing cabinets; take files out of filing cabinets.

Crab: Pretend you are a sea crab. Walk quickly sideways, pretend to munch on others, give quick pretend pinches which make them laugh in delightful surprise. Can be crabs walking sideways, hermit crabs in their shells, a sea urchin that opens and closes, the water flowing in and out, etc.

    Version 1: Everyone does the same creature or element (as announced by the Leader). **Version 2:** Each person does a different creature.

Cracking Up Too Much to Talk: (See "Can't Talk".)

Crazy Hair Laughter: Show off your disheveled, crazy hair. "Can you believe this stuff?"

Crush That Butt Laughter: You are driving and see a lit cigarette butt on the road. You want so much that a nearby car's tires would run over it and put it out. One car misses… another misses (you laugh each time, "Oh well!")… then, a car *does* run over it. "Yay!"

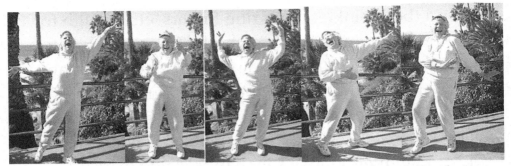

Dances   Everyone laughs for 10-plus seconds while doing a style of dance as announced by the Leader:

Ballet	Flamenco	**Country Line Dancing**
Waltz	Jitterbug	**Belly Dance**
Tango	Salsa	**Hippie/Free Form,** etc.

   Variation: Each person can do their own choice of dance-style - many different dances are happening at the same time.

Darts (Dartboard, Throwing Darts): In two groups. Group 1: Dart Throwers, aiming carefully or tossing with eyes closed, "Another bullseye!" "'Got so close – Aww…" Group 2: Dart Boards, "Oooh, that tickles!" "Good shot, yay!" etc. (These are magnetic darts – no pain!)

Dear Friend Leaving: The other person is a cherished friend who is moving away. Express gratitude, appreciation, and joyful memories with each person.

Defibrillator: Some people are laughing Doctors, others are unhappy Patients. The laughing Doctor puts a defibrillator device to the Patient's chest, and with a shock ("Clear!") they burst out laughing, everyone's hearts full of joy. Exchange roles.

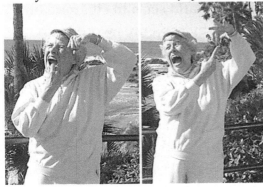

Dentist Laughter: Drill and pull out your own tooth. Hold up the extracted tooth and admire your handiwork. Rinse and repeat.

Die Laughing Sequence

Laugh Yourself to Death: Laugh big and long, eventually collapsing to the ground. Then lie still and quiet for a few seconds. (Can divide into two groups for the following, and switch roles after the "Reincarnation" portion):

Group 1: **Lying in State:** Lying still, laugh at the commotion by the people around you. (While:)

Group 2: **Surrounded by Angels:** Be angels playing harps and floating/flying around, laughing peacefully and angelically.

Reincarnation (also see "Being Born"): Group 1: From the womb, become born and rejoice at discovering life. Group 2: Clap and celebrate as you see the others coming to new life.

Directions: Ask for directions (in gibberish/laughter); one person points one way, another points another way... walk away confused; keep asking others.

Dominos: Everyone sets up rows of dominos (anticipatory "Ha ha ha ha ha's...."). Leader knocks down Domino #1 – all are thrilled and delighted as the rest of the dominos fall over, all around them.

Variation: Everyone sets up rows of dominos all around. Leader knocks down the first domino – but it doesn't work; *none* of the other dominos fall. Everyone laughs: "Oh well; it was fun trying!"

Doctor Jekyll and Mister Hyde: (Variation on "Milkshake".) Pour from one test tube to the second, "Ayyy;" from the second to the first, "Ayyy;" then lean back and drink. **First round**: Become Dr. Jekyll; cerebral, haughty, "holier-than-thou," scoffing. **Second round**: Become Mr. Hyde, a snarly guttural hunkered-over man-beast (like "Lion"). **Third round**: Go back and forth several times between the two characters, switching instantaneously.

Donkey Laugh: Lift head up and back, then forward, braying like a donkey: "*Hee*, haw, *hee*, haw."

Dragons and Knights: In two groups. One group are Dragons, the others are Knights. Dragons play with the knights, flaming them with their breaths, chatting between themselves (in gibberish) how amusing it is to have knights to play with. Knights have fun being "burnt" on their behinds, enjoying the push and pull of the game. Switch roles.

Drinking Song Laughter: Everyone sings a different song (words in gibberish), raising their cups, toasting, laughing and drinking.

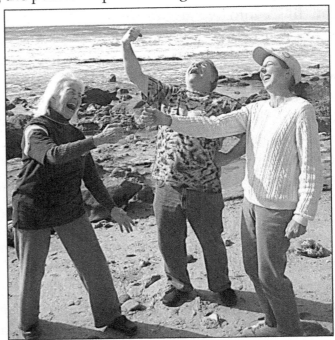

Driving Laughter: Move around as if driving cars or motorbikes. Honk the horn, wave, wink, make arm signals, perhaps a gentle bump…

Drunk Waiter Laughter: Be different people in a restaurant with waiters who are drunk. Have fun laughing (it doesn't really matter) and feeling loose.

 Variation: One or a few people *are* the Drunk Waiters, who walk around dizzily, spilling drinks and food, etc. The rest are very amused and sympathetic customers. Can mix up roles.

Dudley Do Everything ("Mellerdrammer Laughter") sequence
Act out each character and occurrence:

 Heroine (fluttery eyelids, sweet, innocent, hand to forehead).

 Hero (dashing and heroic, puff up chest, devil-may-care, show muscles).

 Villain (twirl moustache, mischievous, snooping).

Two groups: **Imperiled heroine** ("Oh, no!") and **Villain** ("I'm going to tie you to the railroad tracks!"). Switch roles.

Railroad Train ("Choo, choo, hah, hah, whoo whoo") – speed up.

Cavalry to the Rescue! "Ta-ra, ta-ra!" (but they get lost, so:)

Hero Arrives ("Yay!") triumphant.   Villain ("Waah") disappointed. Switch roles.

Hero and Heroine Reunited (Victorious, grateful, "Ha ha!") Hug, celebrate; walk down the wedding aisle, wave at the assembled guests.

E.T. Laughter: You are an extraterrestrial who lands on earth seeing everything for the first time; delighted by whatever you see (and feel, and smell, and hear...). Be sure to touch the others' hearts!

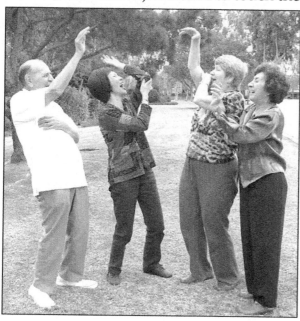

Elephant Laughter: Dangle arm in front of head. Snort up water and spray on each other. Pick up trees with your trunk and lay them down. Be scared by mice.

Elephant Trunk Laughter: Dangle one arm in front of your head to be your trunk. Swing your trunk gently from side to side as you walk with the other arm behind you (it is your tail). Can link arms ("trunk to tail") to make an elephant chain.

"Enjoy your wrinkles!": Show off with accomplishment your smile lines, forehead wrinkles, etc. (can be on arms, belly, knees, anywhere.)

Variation: Enjoy *others'* wrinkles; compliment, praise, "Great smile!"

Escaping Prisoner: Huddled over, move around like you are looking to see if the coast is clear… then burst out joyfully, "I've escaped!"

Evil Laughter (Mad Scientist): Rub your hands in a nasty way and snicker, malevolently. "Bru-ha-ha-ha-ha!"

Evolution Laughter: Be a proto-amphibian; climb out of the primordial soup and take your first breath. Wow!

Exploding Body Parts Laughter: Different body parts "explode" into laughter. Fingers; head; foot; buttocks; ear; tummy; armpit…

Eyes Closed Laughter: (Requires a group comfortable with physical contact.) Close the eyes and walk around carefully. Laugh gingerly, then delightedly whenever you connect with someone.

Farmer in Springtime sequence:
> **Driving a Carriage**, leading a team of horses to the field.
> **Spread Forth the Seed** (change arms). Repeat several times.
> **Watering the Land**
> **Feeling the Warm Sun,** arms wide open, turn around and bask.

Feel the Laughter: Put your hand on your throat, laugh and feel the vibrations. Put your hands on different body parts and feel how they vibrate (if at all) as you laugh into them.

Finger Punchlines: One finger on one hand is a "Comedian" who tells jokes in gibberish. The other hand's fingers are the "Audience" who laugh and wiggle at the "Comedian's" jokes. Can change hands/fingers, telling yourself (your hands) jokes and laughing hysterically
> **Variation**: Walk around finger-joking to *other* peoples' hands, whose fingers laugh-wiggle in response. Trade roles.

86

Fishing (Fisherman's Laughter): Cast out your line; reel it in; repeat; on the third try: you caught something! Reel it in (can struggle) and share with others: a tiny fish, a whale, a shark, a piece of seaweed, an old boot…

Fitness Studio (Fitness Club, Gym) sequence **Exercising** on various devices/equipment.

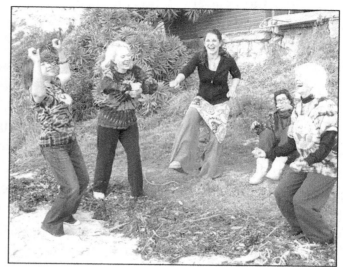

Smell in the locker room = Phew!

Shower, towel yourself dry.

Step on the Weight Scale. Can laugh in accomplishment, or resignation…

Flea Laughter: Pretend your body is covered with fleas biting you. Scratch your fingers all over. See if you can help your itchy neighbors.

Flowing Skirt: You have a long flowing skirt and play with it, swinging in the breeze.

Fly-a-Kite Laughter: With a partner. One is the Kite, the other is the Kite Holder. The Holder will pull, release, shift sides. The Kite sometimes follows, sometimes does not; goes slower, faster, suddenly dips, breaks away free, etc.

Follow the Leader #1: Start in a circle. One person is the "Leader." They do any movement with laughter: any exercise, or any gesture; everyone else copies them. After a few seconds, the person next to them becomes the "Leader" (and everyone else copies the second person). Continue, changing Leaders every five seconds or so until everyone has had a turn.

      Variation: Follow the Leader (Moving Around): Start in a line. One person will be the head of the line. At the command of "Go," this person does a movement, walking ahead and laughing, and everyone copies them. After a few seconds, the first person goes to the rear of the line, and the next person in line becomes the "Leader;" everyone else copies them. Continue, changing Leaders every five seconds or so.

      Variation: Musical Instruments (see "Band/Marching Band".)

      Variation: Follow the Leader (Shadows): Start in a row, with the sun or a bright light behind such that your shadows (hopefully long) can be clearly seen on the ground. The person on one end does a movement while laughing, the others (looking at their shadows on the ground) copy the movement. After a few seconds, pass the "Leader" role to the next person.

Follow the Sport-Leader: One person does the action of a favorite sport (tennis, fishing, baseball, dance, hike, running, bowling, golf, etc.) for five to 10 seconds and everyone else copies them. Go around the circle so everyone has a turn doing the sport and the others copy them.

Food Fight Laughter: Please play with your food! On your marks... get set... throw! (Follow with "Shower - Variation 2" or "Hosing Off" exercise.)

Forgot My Money/Purse: Go shopping for clothes at a fancy boutique/store, get ready to pay: forgot my purse/money!

Fortune Teller (variations)

Palm Reader: Look in your hand and find your Giggle Line; show to others; laugh at what you see in their palm.

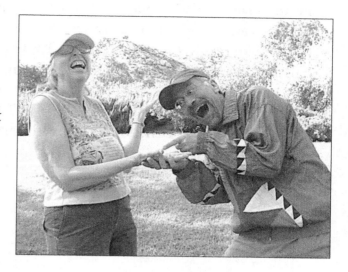

    Variation: When you touch your palm to another person's hand, both of you receive an Electric Jolt of Hilarity.

    Look into the **Crystal Ball**, wondering…? When you see your future, it makes you laugh. Share with others.
    Tarot Card Lay out each card and laugh; share.
    Reading Bumps on someone's head.
    Psychic Mind-Link, hearing spirits, any "psychic" reading.

Found My Glasses Laughter: Lost your eyeglasses; look and look, searching all over for them – and there they are! They were on your forehead all along! Laugh and share with others. (See photo with "There's Your Glasses!")
    Variation: In two groups. Half are seeking their glasses, other half point the glasses out to the seekers – on their own heads.

Freezing Laughter: It's cold outside, everybody's shivering with laughter. Blow "ho-ho-ho's" on hands, slap arms with palms; warm each other up.

Funny Faces: Move around and make funny faces with each person (with good eye contact) and try *not* to laugh. (Follow with an expressive, outgoing laugh like "Hearty" or "One Meter".)

Funny Fries and Silly Sauce: You have a big pile of french-fried potatoes and goopy dipping sauce. Feed yourself, then others. It tastes hysterically funny – and so satisfying! Can also put on head, balance on nose, toss across room, catch and eat on the fly....

Funny Movie Laughter: With a partner (or in two Groups). Person/Group # 1 finds the movie very funny: big laughs. #2 is not amused: polite, half-hearted laughter. Reverse roles.

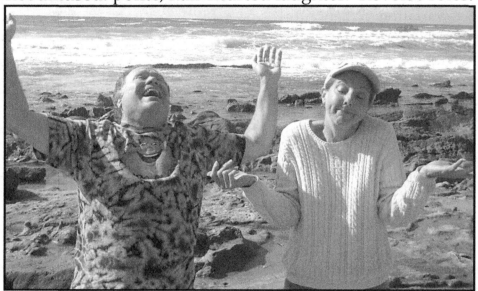

Variation: With a partner. Go back and forth between finding the movie hysterically funny, and barely humorous at all. Try to switch together so that one is always laughing big while the other is laughing small.

Gardening Laughter: Chop the soil with a hoe; dig a hole with a shovel; plant a seed; pour on water. Be the growing plant/flower.

Gelato Laughter: In one hand, hold a cone with a large scoop of gelato. Lick the gelato several times, laughing like a happy young child. On the third lick, the gelato falls off the cone and to the ground. Ha ha ha! With the cone, pick the gelato back up. Resume licking.

    Variation 1: Drop the gelato onto your arm. Lick it off.

    Variation 2: Drop the gelato onto your neighbor's lap... --- Just laugh! (End of exercise!)

Gibberish Punchlines 1, "One-Word" Variation:

In a circle, everyone takes a big inhale together (optionally raising their arms). One person says a single word in gibberish, and all laugh as though the word was incredibly funny (as if that word was the punchline of a fantastic joke). Go around the circle, everyone inhaling deeply together, each person (one at a time) saying a gibberish word, everyone laughing on the outbreath.

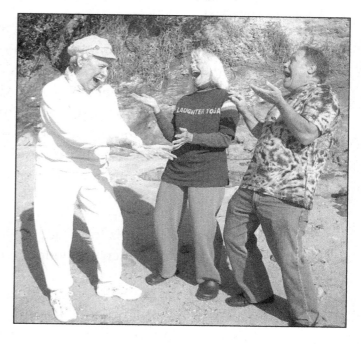

We find this One-Word version is less tiring than the full-on Gibberish Punchlines (where participants may laugh for 10 to 15 seconds after each "joke" and only four or five people can deliver the Punchline before the group starts to get too tired). In this One-Word version, the laugh only lasts as long as one outbreath - about five seconds. Thus, a group as large as 15 or 20 can do the practice, everyone getting a turn, without anyone getting too tired.

Gibberish Punchlines 2, "Gibberish Quips" Variation: One person says a Gibberish Punchline (the last few words of a pretend joke) – everyone laughs *at random*. As if sophisticated British ladies at a highclass Tea Party, participants (in gibberish): make comments to the joke-teller; add to/embellish the joke; make side-comments to each other; and crack up with one another. Continue for 45 seconds, everyone quite delighted with themselves and each other.

Gibberish Punchlines 3, Doggie-style: Deliver the joke in dog-sounds; everyone howls at the punch line.

Gibberish Punchlines Advanced Variations. We call these "Advanced" Laughter Exercises because they first require the ability to laugh *at nothing*. "Words" and "numbers" are used as a trigger, but they are now free of having any meaning.

    4. Punchline Only: One person says the last few words of a joke (in a real language). (Example: "*Now* look how many there are!") Everyone immediately laughs hysterically (even though they don't know the build-up to that particular joke). Many people take a turn.

    5. Laugh at the Numbers: (Based on the notorious "real" joke.) The teller says a number, like "Forty-seven!" and everyone laughs as though it was incredibly funny. Many people have a turn. Can say numbers in different languages, or nonsense ("A gazillion and forty-eleventeen!")

Giggle Molecules: The air is full of giggle molecules. Take in a big, big breath – hold it a bit – then giggle/laugh it out.

Giggling Monks Laughter: Be a row of monks walking to a ritual. Start with a slow Gregorian chant: "Ho, ho, ho ha-a- ha-a hee…" Remember something funny and slowly start giggling, gradually grow into chuckling and big deep laughter.

Going to the Dentist sequence (Also see "Dentist".)
    In the waiting room, nervous.
    A child comes out who has been screaming in pain, and when s/he is gone, all the others **laugh in relief**.
    Someone comes out with their extracted **tooth in a bowl; everyone admires.**
    "It wasn't so bad!"
    Paying the bill (emptying pockets; or signing credit card)

Golf: Giggle nervously getting into position; laugh gently taking practice strokes; big guffaw as you Go For It… look, look, look: A Hole in One!

Good Babysitter Laughter: Comfort the baby; change the diaper; feed the baby; read to the baby; answer the phone with a smile. (Follow with "Bad Babysitter".)

92

Good Hair Day: Wake up, look in the mirror - your hair looks fantastic, like a master hairstylist was working on it all night long! Relish how great you look, show off, enjoy the others' great hair.

Good Witch/Bad Witch: Good Witch blesses with magic wand, dances like a ballet dancer, floating in a bubble, etc. Bad Witch has gnarly fingers, cackles maniacally, throws laughter spells. Can divide into groups, or mix up at will.

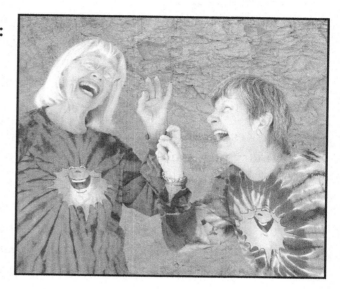

Goofy Kid (Childlike Laughter): Be an innocent, goofy little kid, wearing a half-frozen smile as you chuckle away; can lift shoulders up and down, "Hyuck, hyuck, hyuck!"

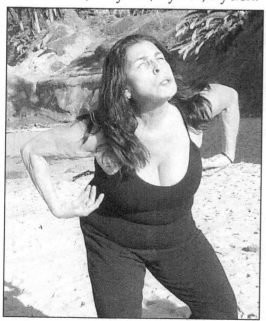

Gorilla Laughter: Romp around like a monkey: flail arms, beat on chest, swing from vines, pick bugs from other's hair (which you eat, or feed to them), peel and feed each other bananas.

Got an "A" (or Got the Job): Open a letter; you got the job you wanted (or the Grade 'A' you hoped for)! Celebrate, congratulate, leap for joy.

Gratitude Laughter: Start with hands to heart. Move around, consciously changing what comes into your awareness: another person, a spot on the wall, your own shoe, a ceiling beam, etc.. Greet it by opening your arms, welcoming it into your heart with grateful laughter. Continue for many items, including people, their clothing, the glint in their eye...

Greek Restaurant Laughter: Some are Belly Dancers, others raise imaginary plates and smash them on the floor. Everybody dance! Drink! Be Merry! *Hopa, ha-ha-ha!*

Guru Laughter: Put one hand on your head as if to say: "I learn from my mistakes, ha ha ha." Put the other hand on your head atop the first hand, as if to say: "I learn from others' mistakes, ha ha ha." Walk around connecting with others, admitting your humility.

Happy Cows: You are a cow. Squeeze your udders – it tickles; squirt some in your face. Walk around squirting each other. (See "Milk Cow".)

Hay Fever: Pick your favorite flower. Bring it to your nose and smell it, and sneeze: "Ha - ha - ha - haa-*choo*!" Repeat several times.

Here Comes the Sun (Sunrise; or Sunrise-Sunset Laughter):

1. Bend low at the knees, arms lay on top of each other just above the head. 2. Slowly lift up, the head rising above the level of the arms (the "horizon"),

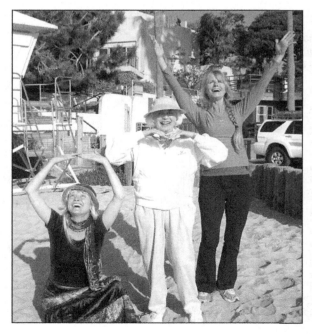

94

laughing as you "peek out" your head (the Sun rises). 3. Grow into a big revealing laugh, shining everywhere (evolve into "Hearty Laughter"). 4. Pull back down – sun is setting. Repeat.

High Five But You Miss: Try to "high-five" someone (a single hand-to-hand slap), but you miss. "Oh well!" Walk around and try to do with many other people, always missing.

High Heels Laughter: Put on high heel shoes and walk all discombobulated and awkwardly.

Hokey Pokey Gibberish: Do the "Hokey Pokey" dance, everyone singing the words in gibberish.

"Honey, We're Pregnant!": Divide into two groups (each with mixed genders). Group 1: "Mothers" who tell husband (in mime, laughter or gibberish) that they are pregnant. "Ha ha ha; surprise!" Group 2: "Fathers" who react to the news (joyfully, despairingly, relieved - whatever) laughing. Switch roles.

Horse Race Laughter: Two groups. #1 = Race horses, at the gate, eager to go. Get ready, then: Take Off, run around laughing! #2 = Spectators, eager for the horses to go. Prepare, then: "They're Off!", cheering, amazed, winning, celebrating. Switch roles.

Hose Laughter: Divide into two groups. In the first group, each person personifies a negative emotion (fear, anger, depression, etc.) and that they are "stuck" in it. With the second group, each person has a Fire Hose of laughter, love and joy to free up the person trapped by the negative emotion. Second group members laugh while spraying/hosing the unhappy persons. The unhappy ones become happy. Switch roles.

Hosing Off: Divide into two groups. First group: each person has a Fire Hose; second group gets hosed clean. Switch roles.

Hug Yourself Laughter: Wrap your arms around you and give yourself a big hug. Can also stroke, pet – and praise! ("I love you! You're my favoritest person in the whole wide world!")

Hula Hoop Laughter: Pretend to be circling a hula hoop around the waist (neck, leg, arms, tongue...).

Hungry Rabbits Laughter: Be rabbits, stealing carrots and greens, hopping away to eat them, coming back for more.

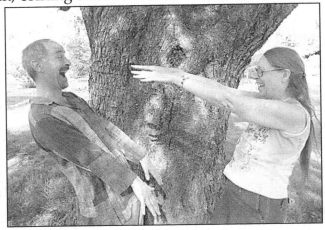

Hypnotism Laughter: Swing (like a pendulum) a hand or arm in front of the face (yours, or others'), taking it all very seriously. Then everybody cracks up! Can hypnotize yourself; try to mesmerize nearby birds or animals, the sun, the wall; walk around like a hypnotized zombie.

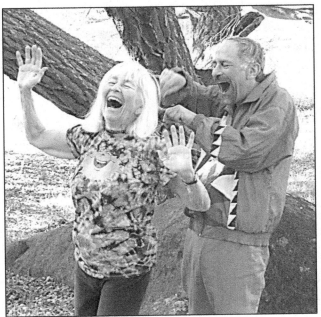

Ice Cube Down the Back: Drop ice cubes down each others' backs; get hysterical, run around trying to remove, help others – or pour in more. Shake yourself up - it feels great!

Incorrigible Kid (Sequel to "Naughty Naughty"): You are the rascally kid who is having the finger waggled at you. Grin sheepishly: "Yeah, I have been a bit naughty – but I am so lovable, you just gotta love me anyway!" Shrug shoulders, giggle.

Proud Parent (or "Gotta Love 'Em!") (Sequel to "Incorrigible Kid"): With a partner. While one person is the "Naughty" Kid, their counterpart is the beaming parent, whose child can do no wrong. "That's my kid, and I love her/him, even when s/he is naughty" or "Aww, isn't s/he great? I just love you, darlin'!" Act proud, boasting to fellow parents; adoringly to the Kid. Switch roles.

Inside Your Head Laughter: With a partner. One person looks in the other's ear; finds stuff (or nothing) and laughs: "So *that's* why you are the way you are!'" The other person laughs with self-acceptance ("Yeah, that's just the way I am!"). Switch roles. (Can walk around changing partners and sometimes be the Looker, and sometimes be the One Whose Head Is Looked Into.)

Isadora Duncan's Demise Laughter: Your long neck scarf gets caught in the wheels of your open-top car; as you choke, you are laughing hysterically at what a ridiculous way to go.

Jeffrey Drinking Water: Just hold a glass, laughing. Passing the time (not actually drinking... well, maybe an occasional sip).

Jellyfish: Move in slow motion like a jellyfish with deep, low, slow laughs. You can "sting" others. Or swoop your arms to float away.

Kaleidoscope Laughter: Looking through a kaleidoscope, turn it around, delighted at the different colors and designs. Share with others.

Kelp Bed (Seaweed and Sea Life):

Half the people are kelp/seaweed. Their feet stay fairly still, the rest of the body sways gently, wrapping around each other. The other half are sea creatures: dolphins, sea lions, sharks, fish, crabs; who swim and weave around the seaweed (and each other). After 20 seconds, exchange roles.

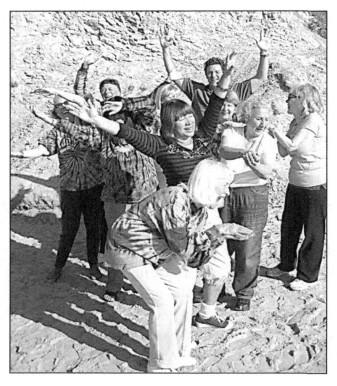

Ketchup Fight Laughter: Squirt, pour, scoop, fling "ketchup" at others; let it ooze down your face, back, into your pants... (It feels great!) Can also do mustard, relish, spaghetti...

Ketchup Laughter: Thump against the end of the pretend ketchup bottle (the ketchup inside is stuck): Once ("Ha..."); Twice (still stuck) ("Ha..."); then it pours out fast all over the sandwich; laugh at the hopeless mess.

Kids-Themed Laughter
    'Don't want to clean up my room (lots of stepping over junk involved).
    Is it really bedtime?
(See also "Playground, Recess/No Recess, School, Test, Got an 'A'," etc.)

98

Kitten Chasing a Butterfly Laughter: Kittens chasing a butterfly are very focused, as they jump, leap, swat, pounce. Rest, and then - get back to it!

Laguna Greeter: You're a grizzled, bearded man who waves greetings to everyone who comes to your village. Bend the knees, make big broad gestures, wave to people both near and far away. Can use both hands. (See also "Waving".)

Laugh at Ourselves (Hold Up a Mirror): Each person goes to another with their hand up, palm flat, as though they were holding a hand mirror, putting it in front of each other - as if to say, "This is who you are". When you look in the mirror you find that you look very funny.

Laugh With Your Hands: Laugh while opening and closing the fingers of the hands, as though the hands were talking to each other. Do hands-to-face, and/or hands-to-hands. Walk around and interact with many people.

Laugh Without Smiling: Keep your lips down or pursed while laughing deep and low. Walk around and laugh with the others without opening the mouth into a grin. (Follow with an outwardly-expressive practice with a big smile such as "Lion Laughter" or "Hearty Laughter".)

Laughter Meditation - Bubbles in your Body Variation (Often done with seniors): Participants sit comfortably with both feet on the floor, close their eyes and imagine soda pop or champagne bubbles coming up through their feet; little tiny bubbles, that are also giggles. Leader says: "Allow the bubbles to flow up your ankles, your calves; as they flow they become bigger, as does your laughter. Allow the laughter bubbles to fill your pelvic girdle, your solar plexus," (more laughter - you as leader will by this time be setting the pace and intensity of the laughter) "and it naturally ebbs and flows, as you progress up through the rib cage, across the shoulders, down the arms to the elbows; elbows to the finger tips, back up and down the spine and finally into the head and out the top of the skull, flowing into an area about two feet all around the body." Speak rather quickly to capture their attention such that no stray thoughts enter the mind of the participant and they can focus only on their experience of relaxation. (Hypnosis-theme suggestions from Dianne McNinch.)

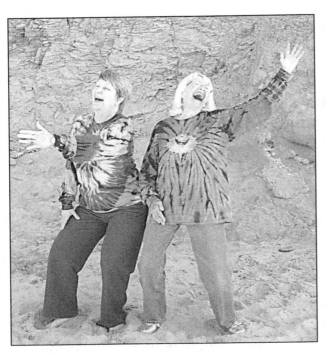

Lawn Sprinklers: Cross one arm in front and towards the opposite side of the body. Imitating a water sprinkler, bounce the arm and hand up and down a few inches as it crosses in front of you and to the other side, saying "Ch- ch- ch– ch- ch- ch- ch..." When the arm gets to its full extension, bring it back across in smooth motion, making a steady-stream laughter sound. 2. Repeat with the other arm. 3. Cross the arms in front, make the "ch-ch-" sound as you uncross and spread the arms wide; laugh as the arms re-cross. 4. Start with the arms wide apart; "Ch-ch-ch-" as they come to the center and then cross; steady laugh as the arms open wide again. 5. Unscrew the hose from the Sprinkler; dash about spraying each other with laughter water.

Let Your Light Shine: At first covered up (as in "Shy Laughter"), then open up and shine! Step forward with pride: your hair looks great, your personality is great; you are radiant! (Similar to "Peacock".)

100

Share your beaming brilliance with others; can give "appreciation" and thumbs-up moves to acknowledge the others' magnificence. (Precede with "Shy Laughter" or "Silent Laughter".)

Light-as-a-Feather Laughter: You are a feather being blown in the wind, or by a fan. Light, airy laughter. You can wave to your fellow feathers as they float by, join them on an airwave.

Lighthouse Laughter: Be a lighthouse, beaming out laughter rays and making foghorn sounds. "Ho---oh; haw----aw."

Limbo Laughter, version 1: Everyone is doing the limbo dance, leaning back (or ducking) under numerous limbo poles. Cheating is welcome!

Limbo Laughter, Version 2: Each person does the limbo, one at a time; two others hold the limbo pole; all the rest cheer them on. Cheating is funny!

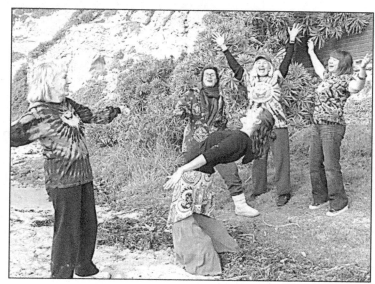

Limerick Gibberish: Say a line in gibberish, others follow. "Tag" someone in gibberish, they tag you back quickly.

Little Dwarves: There are an abundance of little dwarves (elves, gnomes), a few inches tall. Drop them into others' shirt backs (as well as your own); they tickle you as they clamber around inside your clothes.

Long-Lost Friend Laughter: Bump into a friend you haven't seen for 15 years; hug and laugh.

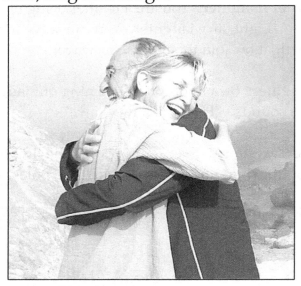

Lost Keys: Finish a three-mile hike. Realize you left your keys at the other end; everyone has to go all the way back. "Oh well - Ha ha ha!"

Love Birds: Be two lovey-dovey birds, cooing and laughing tenderly.
    Variation: Be a whole coop-full of love birds.

Lumberjack Laughter: Chop down a tree. Make a sound (like "Timberrr!"): "Ho -- ho --- ha ha ha ha ha!" Celebrate your success.

Lumberjacks at Play Laughter: Chop down a tree (as above). Catch the falling tree --- and play "Keepaway" with your fellow lumberjacks. (These are very lightweight trees.)

Lumberjack On a Roll Laughter: Walking/balancing on a rolling log (on water). If you fall in, that's just fine!

Make a Quilt: We stitch many pieces of fabric together. Admire it. Then cuddle together under it, cooing with delight.

Making Seaweed Jerky (series): Haul in the seaweed; slice it up; dump it into a bowl. Pour water on it. (Be the seaweed as it slurps up the water.) Pour on seasonings; put it in the oven.

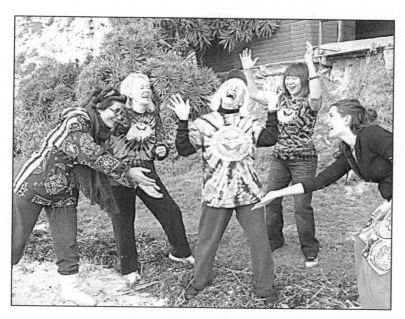

Making Soup: Cauldron in center, everyone chops vegetables and tosses them in to make community soup. One or more people can be "in" the soup; pour broth on self, share with those outside, etc. Yum! (See also "Witches' Brew".)

Making Sweaters: Spin the sheep's wool into yarn. Knit sweaters. Put them on and show off. (Precede with "Sheep and Shepherds".)

Mexican Jumping Beans: Your whole body jumps around. The beans are in your stomach – *it* (your belly) bounces around. The rest of you is surprised and delighted.

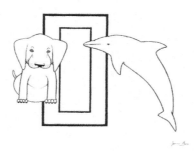

Milk Cow Laughter: One person interlaces fingers with thumbs down, making the cow's udders. The other person grabs the "cow's" thumbs and gently pulls them as if milking. It tickles! Walk around, change roles and partners.

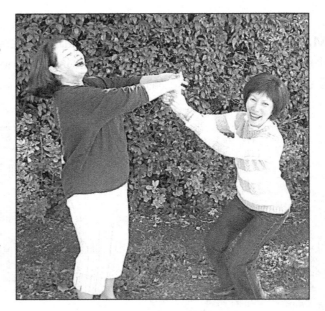

Milkshake Mixer: Drink the milkshake; then shake your body like you *are* the milkshake mixer.

Mirror Laughter: With a partner. Half are Mirror-Hangers, half are Reflections. The Hangers put up the mirror, straighten it, make different faces into the mirror. The Reflections imitate the other's movements and sounds. Switch roles. Change partners. Switch roles again. (Also see "Laugh at Ourselves – Hold up a Mirror".)

Mister Laughter (Spray-Mister): Have a pretend water bottle with sprayer; spray the laughter on yourself and others.

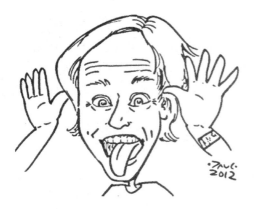

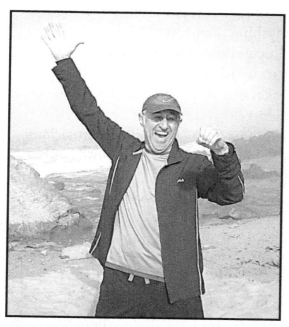

Money Laughter: You get a huge check for teaching Laughter Yoga. You laugh as you receive it, then you laugh all the way to the bank. Then you laugh as you deposit it. Laugh as you look at your checkbook register. (Also see "Jackpot".)

Monster Ball: Portray a movie monster and meet fellow monsters. Can change identities at will. Examples: Wolfman meets Dracula, Frankenstein meets Mummy, etc. Mill around as though at a monster cocktail party.

Monte Python Laughter: Do "Silly Walks" with serious expressions.

Morning Preparations Laughter: Comb your hair; each part of your head has a different laugh-sound. Dry body parts; each has a different sound.

Mountain Climbers' Laughter: Struggling to get up, using ropes and helping one another; together at the top = Victory! "We did it!"

Movie Scenes Act out moments from famous movies.

Casablanca, be the piano player; wink at the guests, laugh to the tune of "As Time Goes By".

Forest Gump (Lawnmower Variation), riding around in a tiny little lawnmower (a small, contained movement); occasionally coming to the crest of a hill and getting louder/faster as you go down the hill, then go back to puttering in "first gear".

Gone With The Wind 1, birthing babies and throwing your hands up to say "I don't know anything about that!"

Gone With The Wind 2, descend the staircase majestically, wearing an elegant gown - made of window curtains.

King Kong peeling clothes off of Fay Wray (and share the pretty, funny little "toy" with others).

Star Wars I, be strange characters in the bar, and/or musicians.

Star Wars II, have a Laser-Saber battle, "be" the sounds of the swords, have a playful swordfight.

Tarzan, swing through trees, pound chest, peel/share bananas, wrestle with alligators/tigers.

(Also see "Singin' in the Rain", "Parade" for the movie "The Music Man".)

Naughty-Naughty with Gibberish: Speaking only in gibberish, walk around and "tell" others several things you have done where you were being "naughty" (laughing all the while).

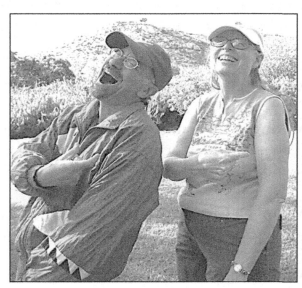

Needle: You get poked with an invisible hypodermic; it fills you with giggle juice. Can inject others with glee.

Nighttime Toilet Visit, version 1: You are a man, you go to relieve yourself – someone left the cover down! Oops --- Ha ha ha ha ha! (This exercise is done by women as well as men.)

Nighttime Toilet Visit, version 2: You are a woman, you go to the toilet – someone left the seat up, you plop down into the water! Whoops --- Ha ha ha ha ha! (Done by men as well as women.)

Nurse's Laughter 1: Stick needles in pretend people. Wrap blood pressure monitor around an arm, pump, take pulse, and look at watch. Write papers. Hold your aching back.

> **Variation:** With a partner. One person is the nurse (doing as above). The other is the patient, laughing at their most amusing nurse. Switch roles.

Nutcracker/Applauding: Divide into two groups. Group #1: Children performing a holiday ballet. Frolic, leap, spin; can also fall down, stub toe, cry, forget what comes next, "steal the stage," etc. Group #2: Parents applauding; sharing their pride with other parents, cheering unconditionally for the kids. Switch roles.

O.C. Girl Accident Laughter: O.C. Girl is driving, talking (laughter/gibberish) on cell phone; car slams into another car, she just keeps talking on the cellphone.

O.C. Girl Driving Laughter: One hand on steering wheel, the other hand applying make-up, checking teeth in the rear-view mirror for lipstick, talking gibberish/laughter on cellphone, etc.

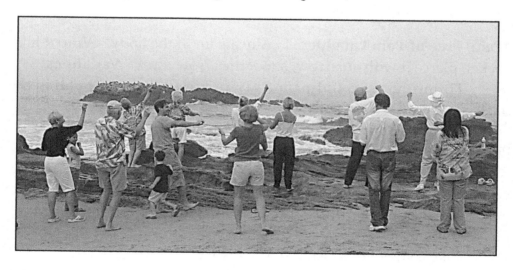

Ocean Wave: Go to the edge of the sea (or lake). Pick a wave and laugh along with it. Build up as the wave grows; burst out laughing as it breaks.

Octopus: Do flowing, underwater–like movements; you're an octopus – moving arms, legs, and additional imaginary arms. Squirt ink to scoot away!

Old Friend: Greet an old friend as if you were both 5-year-olds at Pre-School.

On the Rock Stage: You get to go on stage with the band. Thumbs up: "Aw-right!!!"

One Meter *Schnell!* (also known as "One Meter Laughter after Two Cups of Coffee"): *Done very quickly.* Similar to "One Meter Laughter". Pull hands from 'fingers together' to 'one hand's fingers to one shoulder'; then do the other side; then pull hands apart and bring both arms above head. Repeat many times, all done very fast.

Orchard Laughter: Half are Fruit Trees, half are Pickers. "Ooh, it tickles!" "Yum, this is good fruit!" Switch roles.

Out-The-Nose Laughter: Drinking tea or milk, you laugh so much it comes up and out your nose.

(Pain) Free-of-Pain Laughter: Locate a pain in the body. Wrap it in a packet, pierce it with an arrow, shoot the arrow away. **Variations**:
> **Throw** the **packet-of-pain away**; or **kick** it away; or **put it in the trash** can, etc.
> **Vacuum Cleaner**, suck the pain out of your (and others') body. Put vacuum bag in trash can (or kick it away).
> Say **"Hello" to the Pain, then "Goodbye"**, and wave it off as you send it on vacation (holiday).
> The Pain has a **color; paint a picture** with it. (You can hang the picture for admiration, leave it in a gallery, etc.)
> Take a **shower** – wash the pain away.
> **"Scold" the pain** (talk to it) in Gibberish. (Examples: "Naughty – naughty!" and "How can I help you, sweetie?" etc.)

Palm Reader: (See "Fortune Teller".)

Paparazzi: One (or several) people are "celebrities". The others are paparazzi, autograph hounds, photographers; applauding, asking (in gibberish) for an interview, fawning, praising the "stars," etc.

Parade: Be the instruments in a parade (trombones, flutes, clarinets, tubas, any instrument), the drum major leader, etc. Use gibberish- and laughter- singing. (See "Band – Marching Band".)

Paramedics Sequence (at a weekend Rock Festival)

Give **Artificial Respiration** to a person under the influence of marijuana – mouth to mouth resuscitation, ahah diaphragm work - **become infected** with the marijuana's effects ("stoned").

The Supervisor phones, telling you to assist at an emergency; laughing (**Cellphone** Laughter) because you are stoned and wondering: "Why send *me* to an emergency?"

Hallucinating the paramedics become: Lions; donkeys; pigs; Tarzan...

The Supervisor appears, very angry (**Argument** aka "Naughty-Naughty").

Supervisor orders to laugh not-so-loud (**Silent**).

Supervisor **tries to be serious** (but does not succeed).

Take a big **Shower** to sober up.

Parrot Laughter: Strut around, tilt the head to one side and then another, watch curiously, ask: "'Wanna cracker?"

Pattycake-*Not* Laughter: With a partner. Start to do a handclap game; the other person doesn't know the same version. After hitting and missing for a

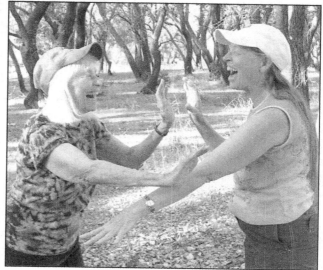

while, toss up your hands: "Oh well, we tried!" Change partners.

Paycheck: Open a letter; it says you got a raise! Show off your new, bigger paycheck. (See "Money", "Jackpot".)

Peacock: (No competition – all peacocks are beautiful) Strut about, genuinely proud of your magnificence, displaying and admiring your own beauty. (Others may cheer for you; you may applaud and celebrate others.)

Pee Laugh: 'Gotta go! Waiting for the toilet, cross your legs anxiously, move around with knees stuck together, smile sheepishly, etc.

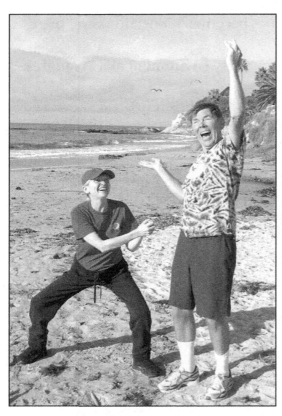

Peel a Banana Laughter, partner version: One person is a banana in a banana skin. The second person peels the skin. #1 is ticklish! #2 is anticipating some fun when the banana is let out. #1 emerges, both are victorious. "Freed at last!"

  Peel a Banana Laughter, solo version: You are inside a banana costume. Peel it off yourself in three or four "undoing-a-zipper" moves; let the skin drop away… and emerge, "Free at last!"

Penguin Laughter:
Turn feet out, hands by sides (palms facing the ground). Walk around like a penguin, spin on one foot; can follow other penguins, bump into them. Variation: Jump into the sea, swim gracefully; then return to the beach and stumble around clumsily.

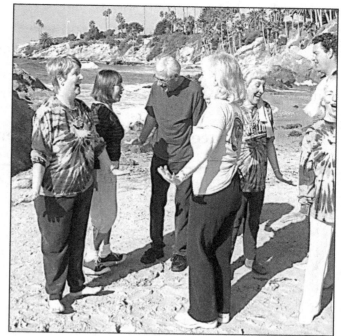

Picking Flowers sequence

  Pick up a bouquet, smell deeply.

  Throw over your shoulder.

  Show to others. When they smell, they laugh.

  Throw to others (abundant bouquets).

  Variation: "Here Comes the Bride": Be Flower Girls/Boys, gamboling in front of the bride, flinging flowers into the air. One person can be The Bride, walking serenely - or crying/giggling nervously - at the rear of the group. Others can be The Father - with or without shotgun, The Groom panicky, Bridesmaids giggling/crying, etc.) (Also see "Smell the Flowers".)

Pie-Eating Contest sequence

  Think about your favorite pie. Everyone is smiling already!

  Pie eating contest is messy; **tie a napkin** under your chin.

  No hands allowed. Put your **hands behind your back**.

  On your mark, get set, go! Put your **face down and eat your pie** as fast as you can.

  Take a break, **raise your head, chew, lick your lips** and laugh.

Face down again to **finish**.

Cheer because "**We have a winner!**"

Wipe off your messy face with your napkin.

Lean back in your chair with a big smile, loosen your belt, rub tummy, "**Ooh, I ate too much!**" (Also see "Upchuckle".)

Pie-In-The-Face (Cheesecake Laughter):

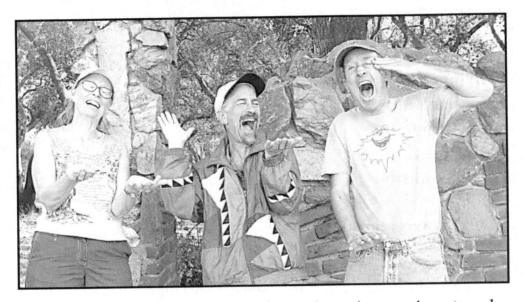

Open a box with a goopy pie; throw imaginary pies at each other. Scoop some off your friend's face, eat a bit… then feed some to them. 'Tastes funny!

Pigeon Poop Laughter: Pigeons are overhead. Duck! They got us; oh well… Wipe imaginary poop off your head & clothes.

Playground: All together, group pretends to be playing in a playground (Leader declares which game, one game at a time). Do three to five games, each game for 10 to 20 seconds):

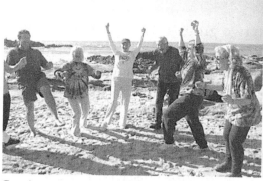 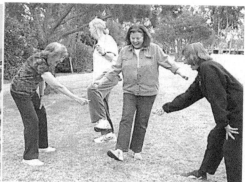

Swinging on Swings (pictured above left), **Jumping Rope** (above right); **Playing with Ball(s)** (below); **Basketball;** **"Catch"; Hop Scotch; Climbing Monkey Bars; Playing with Marbles; Jacks; Teeter-Totter ("See-Saw"**, see "Teeter Totter Laughter"), or others.

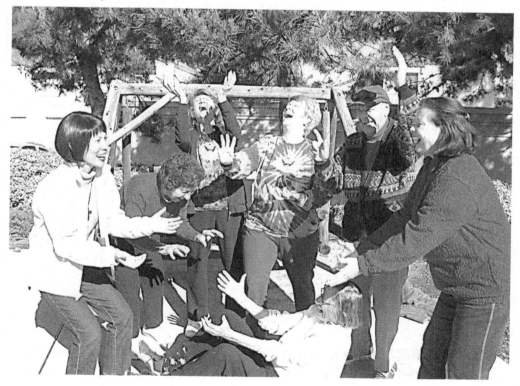

Variation ("Magical Playground"): Leader tells the group that whatever they want to play on magically appears right in front of them at the mere thought of it. Everyone does their own play-games (many different games at the same time). Can change often.

Playground/Admiring: Divide into two groups. Group #1: Children doing playground games (swings, bouncing balls, jump rope, hand clapping games….). Group #2: Admiring/doting parents. Point out your little angel's antics to other "parents," wave at and support your little one, applaud... Switch roles.

Pocket Laughter: Wipe that laugh off your face and put it in your pocket. Walk around with a muffled laugh (lips closed) for a few seconds. Then put the laugh back on your face (open-mouthed laugh). Repeat many times.

Preacher Laughter (Laugh-Evangelist): One person laughs and pontificates (in gibberish) on the virtues of laughing. The others laugh uproariously, applaud, do gibberish "Halleluyah", nod to each other. After ten seconds, switch "Preachers".

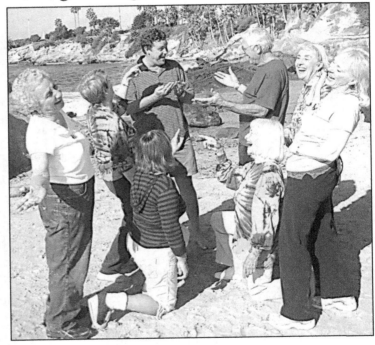

Preying Mantis Laughter: With a partner. One is the female, one is the male. Both do bug-like moves; then the female "bites off the head" of the male, who dies laughing. Switch roles.

Python Laughter: Get strangled by a giant python snake (can be digested, too... and tickle the snake from inside).

    Variation: *Be* the python snake; open your jaws so wide you can swallow another person. *Bon appetit!*

Quiet Laughter: As if someone is sleeping in the adjoining room, laugh very quietly so as to not wake them up. "Shhhh!"

Ran Out of Toilet Paper: Sitting in a public toilet, pulling on the toilet paper roll. It's stuck! Pull one time with sound, "Huh"; pull a second time with "Huh". Pull a third time and it spins free, only to find that there were only two sheets left in the roll. Laugh at this discovery.

Recess/No Recess: The Leader is the schoolground Monitor, who announces: "Okay, kids; time for recess!" All play vigorously for ten seconds. Monitor says, "Stop! No more recess!" Others cry "Boo hoo" for five seconds. Monitor: "Sorry, my mistake: *two more hours* of recess!" Others celebrate "Yay!" and play (20 seconds to several minutes).

Rock-a-Bye Laughter: Lying on the back. Rock the head side to side, laughing gently. Take a big breath in as you center the head; then relax, the head still, and feel the sensations of coming back to balance and quiet.

Rockette Dancing: Everyone gets in a line (arms on shoulders) and "laugh-dances" while kicking up one leg at a time, like flashy Chorus Dancers.

Rock Festival sequence

    Waiting for the Beach Bus, Gibberish talking, move slowly greeting each other due to your morning hangover; wake up your snoring friend.

    Milkshake/special drink (mineral water, sports drink, speedy drink...).

    "**I need to go to the toilet!**"

    Follow the Leader to pass the time.

Drunk walking with a friend.

'Got no money.

Salesman is Drunk - the beer salesman (with a big bottle on the back) has tried too much of the beer; he can't see to pour into your glass.

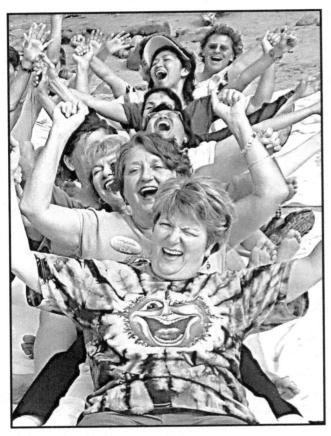

Roller Coaster: Side by side, or seated one in front of the other, or with hands joined. Head up the hill, lean sideways into the corners, lean back, lift hands up for the drops; come back to park. Whew! (Can follow with "Upchuckle, Circus Acts," or create Fairgrounds'-themed rides, attractions, foods, characters.)

'Round the World: Everyone faces in one direction, and sends out a Big Laugh (lasting several seconds). Then *turn around* as your laughs go all the way around the world and hit you from the other direction, slapping you in the front, filling you with even more joy.

Variation: Keep facing the direction where you sent the Laugh; when it comes from around the other side of the world it hits you *from behind*.

Running Through Sprinklers: Frolic, spin and turn as you are passing through the deliciously refreshing sprinkler/fountains of water. Pretend it's the very first time you ever experienced this!

Sample-Eaters Laughter: Be hungry folks scarfing up the free food samples. "Feed at last!"

Sand Fleas: Leap about like little bugs; squeal and nip at each other.

Sandcastle Laughter: You are a sand castle – majestic, yet stiff. Waves come up and dissolve you. What a relief!

Santa Claus: Place hands on your big big belly and let out some hearty "Ho, ho, ho's". Walk around, can bump bellies with other Santa's, give wrapped gifts from a bag...

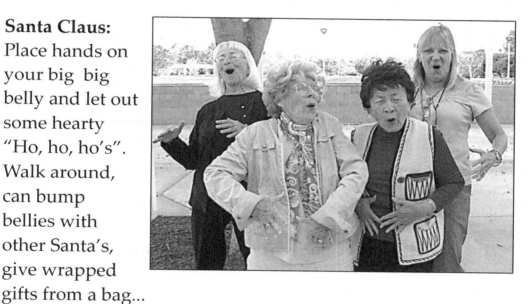

  Variation 1: Carry a big bag of toys; give gifts to everyone.
  Variation 2: In two groups. One group are Santas giving presents to the others. Second group are children: receiving gifts, sharing with each other, giving milk and cookies to the Santas, etc. Switch roles. (Also see "Christmas-themed".)

School of Fish Laughter: The bunch of fish all swim as a group, turning and swooping as closely synchronized as possible.

School Laughter sequence
> **Forgot my homework** ("Oh well!").
> **Missed the soccer kick** (a swing and a miss!).
> **No one wants to sit with me** at lunch. (See "Boo hoo, ha ha" and "Crying Laughter".)

School's Out: Teacher announces: "No school tomorrow!" Everyone leaps in celebration, congratulates each other, plays games like in "Recess" or "Playground".

Sea Lion Laughter: Hands straight down by your sides, wrists flexed. Waddle side to side, legs stiff, lean your body from one side to another, slap arms against thighs while you say, "Ur, ur, urh?"

See the Fun, Goofy Kid Within the Other: You are a five-year-old kid. Look into the eyes and see a friend, who you met yesterday, for the first time, in this new wonderland called Pre-School where you play fun games and do art and crafts all day. "My old friend!" "You're the one who makes those great funny faces!" "I remember you from the sandbox!"

Seaweed and Sea Animals: (See "Kelp Bed".)

Self-Esteem Dial: In your hand you hold a self-esteem meter. If you turn the dial down, you get serious and somber - even sad (laughing all the while). When you turn it up, you feel good about yourself, and get happy. Only you can turn it up (or down).
> **Variation 1:** The dial is installed in your body (you choose where: chest, arm, shoulder, head...). *You* crank it up or down.
> **Variation 2:** You turn it up, and it "breaks" – now, it can only go up - and up and up and up.
> **Variation 3:** *Others* can turn your dial (or push a button), and it only goes up and up and up – each person who touches your Self Esteem Dial (or Button) causes you to become happier and happier and more pleased and confident with yourself.

118

Shampooing the Hair: Washing your hair, then: uh-oh, the water stopped! Exclaim a gibberish profanity ("Aww, orgle-cruk!"); laugh anyway. (Also see "Morning Preparations".)

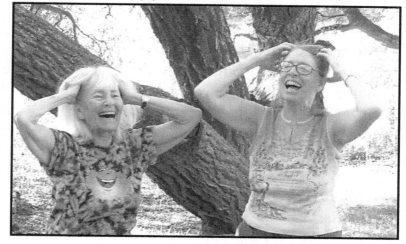

Shapes in the Sand: Draw shapes with your feet in the sand (or on the carpet, on the floor, etc.) "How delightful, what I did!" Draw more shapes. Add on to and change others' shapes - it's all good! Step into your shape, delighted; step into others' fun-filled shapes.

Sharing a Laugh (Snorting): With a partner. Trying to share a laugh, one person 'snorts.' Both bust up laughing even harder. Repeat; try to switch 'snorters' if possible.

She Loves Me, She Loves Me Not: Pick petals from a flower: "Ah ha ha," ("He loves me"- *laugh*); "Ah ha ha ha…" ("He loves me not"- *cry*); repeat three or four times; end with "He loves me, he loves me, *he loves me!*" ("Ah ha ha" three times) - and celebrate!

Sheep and Shepherds: In two groups. Half are sheep, half are shepherds. Shepherds guide and sheer the sheep. Sheep bleat and baah and get tickled. Switch roles. (Follow with "Making Sweaters".)

Sheep Laughter: Be a herd of sheep: Baah-ing, bleeting, sleeping, munching grass.

Shoelace Laughter: Be a child who has tied your own shoelaces, all by yourself, for the very first time in your life. Delighted, joyful and proud; share with everyone around you. "Look, look! I did it; I *did* it!" Also congratulate and be happy for the others – they've done it too!

Shower Laughter (group version): All are in a circle. One (or more) people stand in the center with their eyes closed. The others make thumb-to-middle finger contact with each hand, and interlace their 'finger circle' with their neighbor to each side. All step back, lean down, and say "Aay…" as they step into the center raising their arms. Then step back. Do three times. On the fourth time, after coming in to the center, release hands and laugh while hands are like water showering over (but not touching) the person/s in center (for five to 15 seconds). Change person/s in center and repeat.

  Variation 1 (group): On the fourth time, the outer people gently tap the person/s in the center.

  Variation 2 (solo): Take a shower: turn the water dials; step in ("Oh, it's too cold!" or "Ahh, just right…"); shampoo hair, soap body parts, sing gibberish songs. Rinse off. (Can towel dry.)

Singin' in the Rain: It's raining; dance like Gene Kelly in the famous movie. Open an umbrella, tap dance, swing the umbrella side to side, jump up onto a lamppost, climb up and down curbs, jump into puddles, pretend to be under a spout of water, give the umbrella to someone…

Sinking Boat Laughter: You take your boat onto the lake and see the cork from the bottom of the hull is missing; you will be sinking soon. "Uh–oh. I guess I get to go swimming today!"

Skydiving Sequence Go on a Skydiving trip.

  File **into a bus**, go to airport (nervous and/or anticipatory).

  Exit bus, **put on parachute** and protective gear/clothing.

  Get **into the plane** (anxious, excited).

  Jump out – Wheeee! (thrilled, fearful).

  Drift together to form a star.

  Separate and fly solo; pull ripcord; drift down, **land and celebrate**: you survived

120

Slap Yourself Silly (Give Yourself a Hand): Laugh as you slap/tap all over your own body. Can get quite vigorous. Don't forget your neck and head. (This gentle tapping is beneficial for the lymphatic system.)

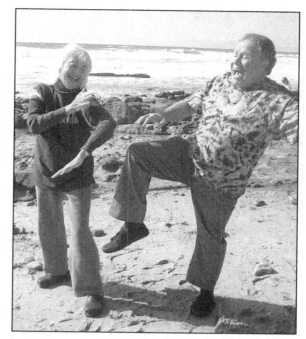

Slow Classical Dance Laughter: Like Isadora Duncan, slow dance movements, pausing as the body forms images as appeared on ancient Greek vases.

　　　Variation: Half are dancers, half are cerebral but appreciative audience.

Slow-Mo Laughter: Move slowly greeting and shaking hands, laugh with low, deep slow-motion sound. Can do Slow-Motion version of any activity: sports, dance, games, etc.

Slow Motion Sports Laughs: Do in slow motion:
Bowling; Football; Throwing telephone poles; Badminton, etc.

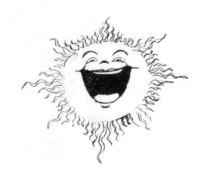

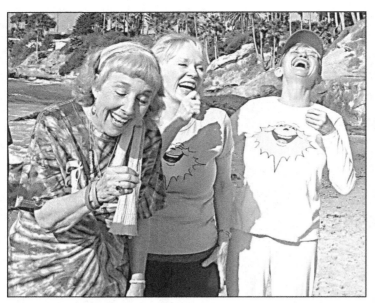

Smell the Flowers: 1. Reach far out ahead of you, grabbing some flowers. 2. Pull them to your nose and take a big whiff (deep breath in). 3. They smell great! Have a big laugh of relief and pleasure. Can be allergic and they make you sneeze-laugh. Can throw them over your shoulder, share your bouquet with others, fling them into the air as you skip around like a Flower Girl at a wedding. (Also see "Pick a Flower".)

Snake Laughter: Hiss, chuckle, rear back; flutter the tongue.

Snoring Laughter 1: Make snoring sounds a whale; like a goat; like an angel, etc.

Snoring Laughter 2: Half the group are Snorers (or fewer – even just one person can be "The Snorer"). The

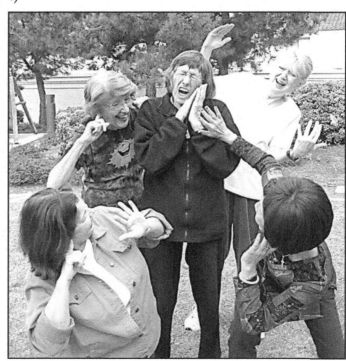

others: plug their ears, throw pillows at the snorer, sing-laugh to cover up the noise, etc. Switch roles.

Snorting Laughter: (See "Sharing a Laugh".)

Space Rocket (very popular in both Austria and Germany): Rub right hand on front of face mask, "Aay…". Then left hand, "Aay…". Repeat each side. Forearms turn, faster and faster, as the engine sound builds up. *Blast Off* - fling arms up as you shoot into space!

Sprinklers: (See "Lawn Sprinklers".)

Spaceship Laughter: You are driving (steering) through space; things shoot by very quickly and everything looks funny!

Square Dance ("Do-Si-Do"): Pair off in couples. Bow to each other, "Allemande Right, Allemande Left," move around, interact with others; clap hands, slap thighs, laugh and connect with each partner.

Standing Ovation: Declare a "Standing Ovation" for someone. Cheer and celebrate. Change the honored one.

Stepped on Chewing Gum: Your foot's stuck! Try to pull it free; circle around the stuck foot; stretch it away – it snaps back. Help!

"Stop Smoking" Series (Instead of being expressed as a negative, "No More Smoking", consider rephrasing as a positive: "Clean Lungs" series or "Happy Lungs" or "Free of Cravings" or "Free from Addictions/Smoking".)
　　　Crying Laughter: You feel conflicted (smoking does give certain good feelings, yet you also want better health and freedom from the cravings). Cry going down, laugh coming up.
　　　Clothes smell bad.
　　　See "No Smoking" sign (disappointed). "I guess I can't go there."
　　　(After finishing the last cigarette): "I'm free! I can do anything, go anywhere, breathe fully! Yay!"
　　　Clothes smell *good*!

See ashtray: "Naughty-Naughty" (waggle finger at the ashtray) and "Forgiveness" (forgive the tray, and others who are still smoking).

See 'No Smoking' sign (liberated). "I can go in there! I can go *everywhere* now! Yay!"

Greet others: "I'm free!" They applaud, share in the celebrating. (Can be in two lines facing each other - a "gauntlet of support," like "Angel Wash".) Each person walks down the center aisle, the others congratulate and applaud. "'Way to go! I knew s/he could do it!" etc. The center person bathes in the joy of their success.

Go into the Woods, and take the deepest breath you have ever taken. It feels *so* good, you cry for Joy!

A note about the "Clean Lungs" (Stop Smoking) Series:
The new exercises were created as a 'challenge,' to be a gift to psychotherapist Eva Lewinsky who served as translator during an advanced Laughter Yoga workshop, and who had expressed a desire to share Laughter Yoga with her patients who wanted to stop smoking. Gabriela Leppelt-Remmel and Jeffrey Briar also wanted to demonstrate how virtually effortless it can be to create new exercises if one is simply open to one's intuition while contemplating a topic. Jeffrey came up with these in seven minutes on the morning of June 6, 2009 (just before the twosome left to deliver the two-day seminar in Hamburg, Germany).

Sunrise Laughter: (See "Here Comes the Sun".)

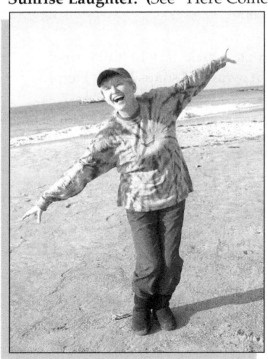

Surfer Laughter:
Swim to the wave, catch it! Ride the board, hang ten; fall in; swim out again. Repeat.

Surfing to Wipeout: You are surfing a really Big Wave to the tune of the song "Wipeout" (Sung as "Hahahahahaha…").

Surprise: (Luck Changes) It's your birthday; you received a gift from your best friend: a single lottery ticket. While scratching the ticket you get the feeling, "Naah, I've never won anything." Then: your ticket is *the winner*; you scream and laugh joyfully, share with others. (Like "Jackpot".)

Swim Strokes: Laugh while doing different styles of swim strokes (Leader demonstrates): Butterfly, Crawl, Breast Stroke, Back Stroke, Dog Paddle… five to 20 seconds per swim stroke.

Taking a Test (Test Laughter): In each hand you have a pile of test papers. Take the top paper from one pile; throw it away over your shoulder, *Hah!* Take the top page from the second pile; throw it away over your shoulder, *Hahaha!* Throw *both* piles of papers in the air; stamp on them on the floor, and celebrate – no more test!

Test, Part 2: It was a class in "Existential Philosophy." The teacher was so impressed with your "No-answer" answer, you got an "A+"! Rejoice, congratulate each other, give high five, dance with joy (like "Got an 'A'").

Tarzan Laughter: (See "Movie Scenes".)

Teeter-Totter (See-Saw) Laughter: With a partner. As you go up, they go down (and vice-versa). Can lean to the sides, or even fall off. (Also see "Playground".)

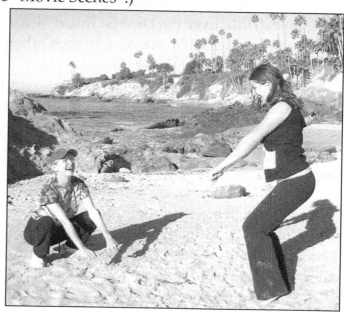

Thanksgiving Theme

Carve the Turkey: Stand and work those carving knives and forks. Pull the stuffing out and put it in a dish. Then cut that bird up; toss the pieces onto the serving platters.

Deep Breath: We want to expand that stomach to make room for our big meal ahead. Breathe in through the nose, and down to the belly. Breathe out through the mouth with a deep contented sigh.

Dessert: It's going to be pumpkin pie with plenty of whipped cream. Spray unreasonable amounts of cream on the pie; spray some on your finger and lick it off. Spray some in your mouth, giggle with the mouth full; turn into a whipped cream spraying frenzy.

Football Game: Intently watching the Big Game on TV; lean forward, side-to-side to watch the moves, with nervous laughter (similar to "Roller Coaster"); the team makes a touchdown! Throw arms up in celebration; give high five near-misses.

Happy Turkey Strut: Be the happy turkey that lived with the vegetarian family - strutting, gobbling, and laughing because you're not going to be eaten.

Hunting the Turkey: Imitate Elmer Fudd on hunting day. To the tune of "Ride of the Valkyrie" (aka "Kill the Rabbit") but using "Ha, ha, ha-ha", "Ho, ho, ho-ho." Walk around as if hunting, stalking the prey, turning quickly to aim the gun in different directions.

Joyful Talk over the Dinner Table: React to funny gibberish stories at the dinner table, nodding to each other, passing imaginary dishes, scooping out helpings.

Morning Stretch: Get up very early to put that turkey in the oven; we need to stretch first. Stretch up and out and down.

Oh-My-Aching-Stomach: Wow! What a great meal! But now my tummy hurts. Walk around holding stomachs, and do a moaning laugh.

Pat That Belly: Pat your stomach in anticipation of the good dinner that you'll be enjoying soon.

Potato Mashing: (Standing or seated.) Mash a big bowl of potatoes with one of those old-fashioned potato mashers (pre-electric beaters). Get rid of all of those lumps.

Stuffing Laugh: Like a chipmunk with its cheeks stuffed with

126

food. Do a humming laugh with puffy cheeks and mouths closed.

Turkey Waddle Laugh: Turkey waddling, gobbling, flapping their wings.

Turkey Wattle Laugh: (That thing that hangs down under their chin is the turkey's "wattle".) Put hand under the chin and wiggle it like a turkey wattle; waddle, gobble and laugh.

--- ---

There's Your Glasses!:
Half the group are looking everywhere for their glasses (nervous laughter). Other half start giggling (four seconds): "I think I know how to find them…" Then: "There they are, right on your head!"

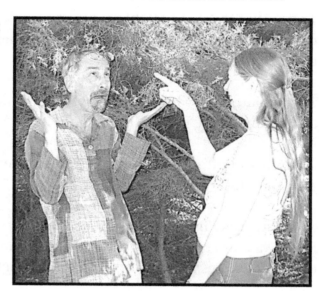

Everyone laughs (Seekers: "Silly me!" The others: "Isn't life weird? I've lost things in my life, too…"). Switch roles. (See variation under "Found My Glasses".)

Tickle Attack: Tickle yourself, anywhere and everywhere; wherever you tickle makes you laugh crazily. Show others where you've found your magic tickle-spots. They can try that spot on themselves.

Tidepool: Pretend to be different tide pool creatures: crab, anenomes, seaweed, octopus, seashell, etc. (Also see "Kelp Bed".)

Tied My Shoelaces: (See "Shoelace Laughter".)

Toy Box Laughter: In the center is a giant box of toys. One person pulls out an imaginary toy and shows how to play with it; everyone else laughs and cheers, "Ooo's and Ahh's."

Variation 1: As soon as the outside people realize what the toy is, an identical toy appears in their hands; play with it (share/interact with others).

Variation 2: Everyone can reach into the center and pull out toys, play and share: a toy-playing frenzy!

Trying-to-Do-Yoga Laughter: Attempt to do some difficult yoga move, like putting your leg behind your head (or even just touch your toes). "I just can't do it!"

Turtle Laughter: Move very slowly with a deep, low laugh: "I've got all the time in the world: Ho... ho... ho...".

Two Cats Fighting Laughter: With a partner. Snarl, hiss, swat. Run away and fight with others.

Two Puppies Fighting Laughter: With a partner. Bark, feint, chase. Run away and come back. Roll on the ground together and just lie there sometimes. **Variation**: Be a whole pack of puppies.

Two Puppies Tug-Of-War: With a partner. Be two puppies playing with a rope in your teeth.

Two-gether Greeters: (Requires participants to be comfortable touching another person.) Two people link up as greeters; they link one arm with the other person's arm (or hold hands, or put one arm on the other's shoulder, or etc.); with the free arm and hand they wave in greeting (to other people, animals, plants, the environment, etc.).

United Nations: Each person speaks gibberish and laughter in the style of a foreign language (which they do not actually speak): "pretend-Chinese", "pretend-Italian", or other, using lots of hand gestures, bowing, etc.

Version 1: Leader demonstrates one laugh-language; everyone walks around talking/laughing with each other in the same language. Repeat with three or more "languages".

Version 2: Everyone picks their favorite gibberish language (or several), and all walk around gibberish talk/laughing in all-different languages.

Universal Laughter: Be floating in space: planets, suns, satellites, stars, comets; you can go super-nova! Or be a Black Hole and absorb everyone. Whoops, watch out for that space ship zipping by...

Unmoving: Try to laugh without moving your face or lips. (Follow with an expressive exercise like "Lion" or "Hearty".)

Up-Chuckle (Heave Ho, or Heave Ho-ho-ho Laughter):

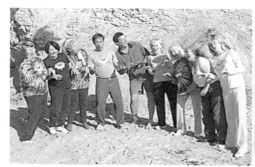 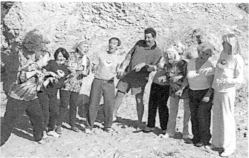

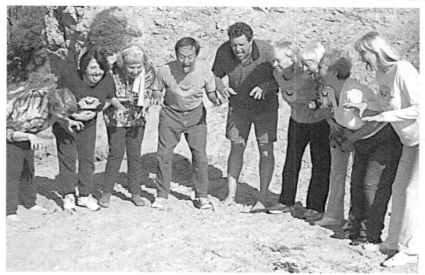

Standing at the side-rail of a ship in troubled seas. Lean to one side, saying "Ay---;" lean to the other side, "Ay---;" then center and "Bleah – ha- ha- ha- ha- ha!" spew out laughter to the ocean below you. Spread face wide and stick tongue way out for the most fun and best benefit to thyroid and parathyroid glands. Repeat several times.

Upside-Down Laughter: Begin standing. Bend over at the waist; look between your legs (or under your arm) and see the world turned upside down. Walk around (if you can) enjoying the funny, inverted world.

Visitor to Laughter Club: You are a stranger who finds the Laughter Club, and you join in; try to laugh louder than the rest of the group.

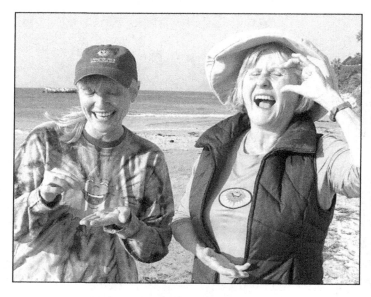

Vitamin Laughter: Open the bottle, take out a vitamin, chew it up and laugh. Take a time-release capsule (for a later laugh). Hey, it happened already!

Vowel Movement: In a circle (hands holding or not). All come toward the center, raising arms while saying a vowel sound, turning into laughter. After the sounds, step back out. Repeat movement with the next vowel sound. Example in English: A (as in "say"); E (like "free"); I (like "high"); O (like "ho"); U (like "hoo"); Y (like "sky")

  Variation 1: Start with the vowel sound, then just laugh.

  Variation 2: Start with the vowel sound; then have the laughter sound be a laugh which is an extension of the vowel. Example: A = Hay hay hay hay hay, E = Hee hee hee hee hee; I = High yi yi yi yi, O = Ho ho ho ho ho, U = Hoo hoo hoo hoo hoo, Y = Why – yiy yiy yiy yiy.

130

Variations: Use the vowel sounds of different languages. (Invite participants who speak other languages to lead the sounds to begin; the others copy them.)

Walk/Talk Like a Seal: (See "Sea Lion".)

Walking a Tightrope: (With Audience) One person walks the rope while others are the cheering, admiring, applauding spectators. Take turns being the walker. Each walker does variations: walk backwards, turn and spin, fall off and fly away, carry another person on your back, use a balance beam, juggle, ride a bike, etc. (See photo with "Circus Laughter".)

Wave (Laughter Wave): Form a circle. The group *is* a wave, forming and breaking. Clasp hands, swoop down to the center, lift arms upward and let the wave break with hearty laughter. Repeat. (Also see "Ocean Wave".)

Waving: Lift one arm, show your palm; wave "Hello" to others (near and far), wave to things all around (door knobs, 'Exit' signs, spots on the wall...) Can use two hands (...perhaps your feet?). (Also see "Laguna Greeter".)

Weight Lifter: Show your muscles, take poses; lift big heavy weights yet scoff at "how easy it is" for you (or be tickle-scared that you can't finish the lift), etc. (Also see "Fitness Studio".)

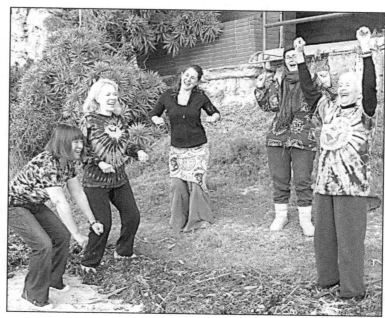

What Happens in Vegas: Cover eyes with hands. Walk around and "wake up" by opening hands and see who you married last night. (!) Express surprise, delight, relief, etc.

Where Babies Come From: Divide into two groups. Group 1 = Cabbages in a patch, eagerly awaiting the storks' delivery. Group 2 = Storks who fly in with babies to place by the delighted cabbages. Switch roles.

"Where's My Glasses?": (See "There's Your Glasses!")

"Where's Our Son?": Look at clock by the head of the bed. Poke partner in side. ("Our son's not here, is he?" Ha ha ha!)

Witches' Brew: Cauldron in center, everyone throws in strange things (toads, body parts, nasty herbs - named in gibberish), cackles with delight, amazed/tickled by the others' contributions.

Wizard and Apprentice: With a Partner. Wizard does magical spell in gibberish and flails arms; Apprentice transforms into something (a toad, broom, handsome prince, cackling witch – Apprentice's choice). Wizard is pleased. Switch roles.

    Variation: In a group. One person is the Wizard, and says "I turn you all into…" (Wizard's choice: gibberish words, toads, trees, stone, water, fire, pickup trucks…). Everyone laughingly becomes that thing. Let several take a turn at being the Wizard.

Wizards and Statues:

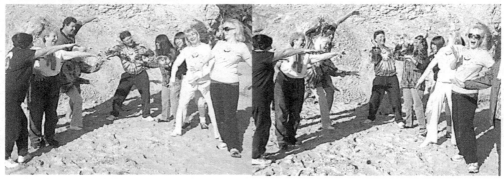

In two groups. One group = nervously giggling "frozen" Statues, ready to come to life. Other group = Wizards. Action: Wizards do gibberish magical spells, flail arms at Statues. Statues come to life and celebrate that they can move. Wizards laugh in satisfaction, admire Statues, congratulate each other. Switch roles.

Wrong Room!, version 1: Everyone is a Woman, who accidentally went into the Men's restroom. Hide your eyes, apologize. Act shocked at what you see – and "where" you see it!
   Variation: Half are Women, half are Men (do not have to be true to their actual physical gender).

Wrong Room!, version 2: Everyone is a Man, who accidentally went into the Ladies' restroom. Hide your eyes, apologize – act shocked at what you see – and "where" you see it. (!)
   Variation: Half are Men, half are Women (the role they play need not be their actual gender).

- END -

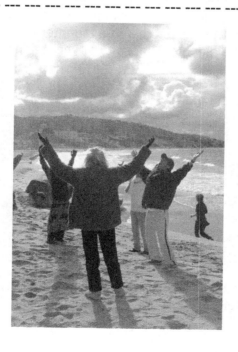

Creating New Laughter Exercises

Imagine the physical expression of any job, hobby, practice or activity. Then *perform* that action, and laugh while doing so.

You can be:

- Flipping pancakes while laughing
- Milking a llama while laughing
- Hitting a baseball laughing
- Driving bumper cars laughing (no matter what happens)…

Any activity can be performed laughingly.

-------- -------- --------

Acknowledgments ~ *Thank You!*

Known contributors to this collection include: Lilia Abreu, Joyce Alderson, Claudia Birck, Jeffrey Briar, Kathryn Burns, Ross Costa, Bill Gee, Sebastien Gendry, Ruthe Gluckson, Cindy Gudel, Joy Hardin, Gail Hunter, Gabriella Leppelt-Remmel, Madan Kataria, Madhuri Kataria, Sparkie Lovejoy, Leigh Meredith, Dianne McNinch, Dawn Passaro, Kevin Roberts, Fiona Skye, Sue Snyder, David Sullenger, Steve Wilson… and undoubtedly others. Sincere apologies to anyone whose name is not mentioned yet who believes they made up an exercise included in this volume. We have often found that when someone thinks they have created a laughter exercise, it already exists somewhere else on the planet. Thanks to all for sharing, and let's keep creating!

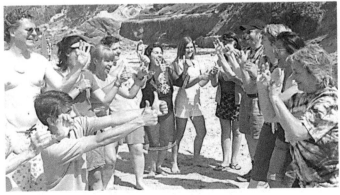

Many of these exercises can be seen in brief videos on YouTube under account names "JoyfulGent" and "Jeffrey Briar".

The Laughter Exercise Session

Formats for Laughter Sessions vary worldwide, but in general we always want to have: a warm-up; 15 to 20 minutes of Laughter; Relaxation; and a wish for Peace. Following is the structure of a typical Laughter Exercise session.

1. Welcome: Advise participants they are to experience "No New Pain". They can always modify any practice to fit their comfort level, or sit it out.

2. Body Warm-Up: We prepare for expressing ourselves with an all-over physical warm-up lasting three to ten minutes, composed of easy stretches and vocalizations. (A video of a simple 5-minute warm-up can be seen at http://lyinstitute.org/the-laughter-club-experience.)

3. Breathing Exercises (pp. 53-56): Do one or two, then repeat the same Breathing Exercise(s) with laughter on the exhalation.

4. Laughter Exercises (15-20 minutes):
> Greeting (Namaste &/or Handshake);
> "Ho, ho, ha-ha-ha" (p.57);
> two Exercises (ending each with "Ho, Ho, ha-ha-ha");
> one Exercise; "Very Good, Very Good, Yay!" (p. 60);
> one Exercise; an easy Stretch/Breathing exercise;
> six to eight more Laughter Exercises, interspersed with "Very Good, Very Good, Yay!", "Ho, Ho, ha-ha-ha", and other easy Stretches/Breathing exercises.

5. Positive Affirmations: The Leader declares something like "We are the healthiest people in the world!" and the others respond with a vigorous cheer: "Yay!" Then say two other affirmations (e.g., "We are the happiest people in the world!" "We love to laugh!" "We are having fun!" "We love everybody!" etc.) each followed by the group cheer.

6. Laughter Meditation (p. 58).

7. Guided Relaxation (p. 59).

8. Wish for Peace; Announcements.

Choosing the Best Exercises for Your Group

Select practices to best suit the participants. For a room full of energetic 7-year-olds you might offer different exercises than if you have a group of wheelchair-bound seniors.

Be considerate of their abilities. Elders usually do not like to get down on the floor, as they find it difficult to get back up; sports-lovers and children may require physically challenging activities to avoid boredom. For initial sessions you might choose exercises that relate to the participants' real lives: people in business enjoy Cellphone and Jackpot; athletic folks like to laugh with sports victories; most adults relate well to Credit Card Bill – the same exercise could be renamed "Report Card" for school-aged children.

After a few sessions - when they trust your leadership and feel comfortable with one another -you can probably expand into any and all Laughter Exercises. Yes, you *can* have your stuffed-shirt business colleagues go to the Playground, stick out their tongues like Lions, and waddle around like Penguins. Trust your intuition, have fun - and share it!

Here are some Laughter Exercises suggested for specific groups:

Children under 13: Lion, Penguin, Bird, Playground, Naughty-Naughty, One-Word Gibberish Punchlines, Hot Soup, Shy, Hearty, American Cowboy, Appreciation.

Well-Dressed Ladies: Cellphone, Laughter Cream, Royal, Appreciation, Milkshake, Naughty-Naughty, Shy, Let Your Light Shine, Laugh at Yourself, Forgiveness, Silent, Gibberish Punchlines 2 (Quips).

Serious Adults (business professionals): Handshake, One Meter, Cellphone, Milkshake, Credit Card Bill, Jackpot, Motorbike, Gibberish Punchlines, Silent, Hearty.

Seniors: Royal, Laughter Cream, Appreciation, Milkshake, Cellphone (Telephone), Laughter Center, Laugh at Yourself, Vowels.

-END-

Encyclopedia of Laughter Exercises (Part 2 of *Laughter Exercises: The Great Big Anthology*)

Compilation Volume:

Laughter Exercises: The Great Big Anthology

(with 120 photographs)

Part 1: Dr. Kataria's Foundation Exercises
Part 2: Encyclopedia of Laughter Exercises

ISBN-13: 978-1533456328

ISBN-10: 1533456321

Black & White Edition, revised & updated 2017

www.LYInstitute.org

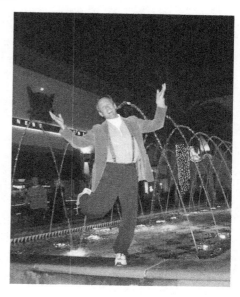

-- Jeffrey Briar

Made in the USA
Monee, IL
24 June 2020

34499317R00079